GERIATRICS *At Your* FINGERTIPS

2003, 5th EDITION

GERIATRICS *At Your* FINGERTIPS

2003, 5th EDITION

AUTHORS:

David B. Reuben, MD

Keela A. Herr, PhD, RN

James T. Pacala, MD, MS

Bruce G. Pollock, MD, PhD

Jane F. Potter, MD

Todd P. Semla, MS, PharmD

PUBLISHED BY BLACKWELL PUBLISHING, INC.
MALDEN, MA, USA

This publication was prepared by Blackwell Publishing, Inc., at the direction of the American Geriatrics Society as a service to health care providers involved in the care of older persons.

Although *Geriatrics At Your Fingertips* is distributed by various companies in the health care field, it is independently prepared and published. All decisions regarding its content are solely the responsibility of the authors. Their decisions are not subject to any form of approval by other interests or organizations.

Some recommendations in this publication suggest the use of agents for purposes or in dosages other than those recommended in product labeling. Such recommendations are based on reports in peer-reviewed publications and are not based on or influenced by any material or advice from pharmaceutical or health care product manufacturers.

Citation: Reuben DB, Herr K, Pacala JT, *et al. Geriatrics At Your Fingertips: 2003, 5th Edition.*
Malden, MA: Blackwell Publishing, Inc., for the American Geriatrics Society; 2003.

ISBN 1-4051-0337-X
Library of Congress Catalog Card Number 2002152770
Printed in the U.S.A.

TABLE OF CONTENTS

AUTHORS

David B. Reuben, MD
Director, Multicampus Program in Geriatric Medicine and Gerontology
Chief, Division of Geriatrics
Professor of Medicine
David Geffen School of Medicine at UCLA
Los Angeles, CA

Keela A. Herr, PhD, RN
Professor
Chair, Adult and Gerontological Nursing
College of Nursing
The University of Iowa
Iowa City, IA

James T. Pacala, MD, MS
Associate Professor and Vice Chair for Medical Student Affairs
Distinguished Teaching Professor
Department of Family Practice and Community Health
University of Minnesota School of Medicine
Minneapolis, MN

Bruce G. Pollock, MD, PhD
Professor of Psychiatry, Pharmacology, and Pharmaceutical Sciences
Chief, Academic Division of Geriatrics and Neuropsychiatry
Department of Psychiatry, University of Pittsburgh
Pittsburgh, PA

Jane F. Potter, MD
Chief, Section of Geriatrics and Gerontology
Harris Professor of Geriatric Medicine
University of Nebraska Medical Center
Omaha, NE

Todd P. Semla, MS, PharmD
Department of Psychiatry and Behavioral Sciences
Evanston Northwestern Healthcare
Evanston, IL
Clinical Assistant Professor
Section of Geriatric Medicine
College of Medicine
University of Illinois at Chicago
Chicago, IL

ABBREVIATIONS

ABG	arterial blood gas
ACC	American College of Cardiology
ACE	angiotensin-converting enzyme
ACIP	Advisory Committee on Immunization Practices
ACOG	American College of Obstetrics and Gynecology
ACR	American College of Rheumatology
AD	Alzheimer's disease
ADA	American Diabetes Association
ADLs	activities of daily living
AFB	acid-fast bacillus
AHA	American Heart Association
AHCPR	Agency for Health Care Policy and Research (now, Agency for Healthcare Research and Quality)
AIDS	acquired immune deficiency syndrome
AIMS	Abnormal Involuntary Movement Scale
ALT	alanine aminotransferase
APAP	acetaminophen
ASA	acetylsalicylic acid or aspirin
ASA class	American Society of Anesthesiologists grading scale for surgical patients
ATA	American Thyroid Association
ATS	American Thoracic Society
AUA	American Urological Association
BIPAP	bilevel positive airway pressure
BMD	bone mineral density
BMI	body mass index
BP	blood pressure
BPH	benign prostatic hyperplasia
BUN	blood urea nitrogen
C&S	culture and sensitivity
CABG	coronary artery bypass graft
CAD	coronary artery disease
CAPD	central auditory processing disorder
CBC	complete blood cell count
CBT	cognitive behavior therapy
cfu	colony-forming unit
CHD	coronary heart disease
CHF	congestive heart failure
CI	confidence interval
CMS	Centers for Medicare and Medicaid Services (formerly, US Health Care Financing Administration, or HCFA)
CNS	central nervous system
COPD	chronic obstructive pulmonary disease
CPAP	continuous positive airway pressure
CPK	creatine phosphokinase

CPR	cardiopulmonary resuscitation
Cr	creatinine
CrCl	creatinine clearance
CT	computed tomography
CXR	chest x-ray
CYP	cytochrome P-450
D&C	dilation and curettage
D5W	dextrose 5% in water
DBP	diastolic blood pressure
D/C	discontinue
DHIC	detrusor hyperactivity with impaired contractility
DSM-IV	*Diagnostic and Statistical Manual of Mental Disorders*, 4th ed. (Washington, DC: American Psychiatric Association; 1994)
DTR	deep-tendon reflex
DVT	deep-vein thrombosis
ECF	extracellular fluid
ECG	electrocardiogram, electrocardiography
EF	ejection fraction
EPS	extrapyramidal symptoms
ESR	erythrocyte sedimentation rate
FDA	Food and Drug Administration
FEV_1	forced expiratory volume in 1 second
FOBT	fecal occult blood test
FVC	forced vital capacity
GAD	generalized anxiety disorder
GDS	Geriatric Depression Scale
GERD	gastroesophageal reflux disease
GFR	glomerular filtration rate
GI	gastrointestinal
GU	genitourinary
Hb	hemoglobin
HbA_{1c}	glycosylated hemoglobin
HCFA	*See* CMS
HCTZ	hydrochlorothiazide
HDL	high-density lipoprotein
HR	heart rate
HRT	hormone replacement therapy
HTN	hypertension
hx	history
IADLs	instrumental activities of daily living
IBW	ideal body weight
INH	isoniazid
INR	international normalized ratio
IOP	intraocular pressure
IPC	intermittent pneumatic compression
JNC-VI	Sixth Joint National Committee on Prevention, Detection, Evaluation, and Treatment of High Blood Pressure
K^+	potassium ion

LBW	lean body weight
LDL	low-density lipoprotein
LDUH	low-dose unfractionated heparin
LFT	liver function test
LMWH	low-molecular-weight heparin
LVH	left ventricular hypertrophy
MAOI	monoamine oxidase inhibitor
MI	myocardial infarction
MMSE	Folstein's Mini–Mental State Examination
MSE	mental status examination
MRI	magnetic resonance imaging
NG	nasogastric
NSAIDs	nonsteroidal anti-inflammatory drugs
NPH	neutral protamine Hagedorn (insulin)
OCD	obsessive-compulsive disorder
OGTT	oral glucose tolerance test
OT	occupational therapy
PE	pulmonary embolism
PEF	peak expiratory flow
PET	positron emission tomography
PNS	peripheral nervous system
POMA	Performance-Oriented Mobility Assessment
PPD	purified protein derivative (of tuberculin)
PSA	prostate-specific antigen
PT	prothrombin time *or* physical therapy
PTCA	percutaneous transluminal coronary angioplasty
PTT	partial thromboplastin time
PUVA	psoralen plus ultraviolet light of A wavelength
QT_c	QT (cardiac output) corrected for heart rate
RBC	ranitidine bismuth citrate *or* red blood cells
sats	saturations
SD	standard deviation
SBP	systolic blood pressure
SIADH	syndrome of inappropriate secretion of antidiuretic hormone
SOB	shortness of breath
SPECT	single-photon emission computed tomography
SPEP	serum protein electrophoresis
SSRIs	selective serotonin-reuptake inhibitors
TCA	tricyclic antidepressant
TD	tardive dyskinesia
TDD	telephone device for the deaf
TG	triglycerides
TIA	transient ischemic attack
TSG	thyroid-stimulating globulin
TSH	thyroid-stimulating hormone
TTP	thrombotic thrombocytopenic purpura
TUIP	transurethral incision of the prostate
TURP	transurethral resection of the prostate

U	unit(s)
UA	urinalysis
UI	urinary incontinence
UV	ultraviolet
VIN	vulvar intraepithelial neoplasia
WHO	World Health Organization
wt	weight

Drug Prescribing and Elimination

Drugs are listed by generic names; trade names are in *italics*. Check marks ($\checkmark$) indicate drugs preferred for treating older persons. Formulations are bracketed and expressed in milligrams (mg) unless otherwise specified. Abbreviations for dosing, formulations, and route of elimination are defined below.

ac	before meals
bid	twice a day
C	capsule, caplet
conc	concentrate
CR	controlled release
cre	cream
ChT	chewable tablet
d	day(s)
ER	extended release
F	fecal elimination
gran	granules
h	hour(s)
hs	at bedtime
IM	intramuscular(ly)
Inj	injectable(s)
IT	intrathecal(ly)
IV	intravenous(ly)
K	renal elimination
L	hepatic elimination
lot	lotion
max	maximum
MDI	metered-dose inhaler
min	minute(s)
mo	month(s)
npo	nothing by mouth
NS	normal saline
oint	ointment
OTC	over-the-counter
pc	after a meal
pk	pack, packet
po	by mouth
pr	per rectum

prn	as needed
pwd	powder
qam	every morning
qd	every day
qhs	each bedtime
qid	four times a day
qod	every other day
S	liquid (includes concentrate, elixir, solution, suspension, syrup, tincture)
SC	subcutaneousl(ly)
sec	second(s)
shp	shampoo
sl	according to the rules
sol	solution
Sp	suppository
spr	spray(s)
SR	sustained release
sus	suspension
syr	syrup
T	tablet
tinc	tincture
tid	three times a day
TR	timed release
wk	week(s)
yr	year(s)

INTRODUCTION

Providing high-quality medical care for older persons requires a special set of knowledge, clinical skills, and attitudes. Many resources contain current, accurate information on evaluation and management of the older patient. However, few are portable enough to be used in the examining room, on nursing home or hospital rounds, or when the clinician is on call outside the office.

In 1998, the American Geriatrics Society (AGS) first published *Geriatrics At Your Fingertips* (*GAYF*), a pocket guide that provides immediate access to specific information needed to care for older persons in various health care settings. The response was extraordinary, and *GAYF* soon became the society's best-selling publication. During the past year, the AGS has created new platforms for *GAYF* to take advantage of the expanding integration of electronic mediums into clinical practice. Specifically, beginning in 2002, *GAYF* became available on the Internet (http://www.geriatricsatyourfingertips.org). With this fifth edition, *GAYF* will take the major step of being available in Palm and Windows CE operating systems. Now, clinicians will be able to have *GAYF* instantly available on their PDAs.

In this edition, we have updated information throughout the text and tables, including recommended diagnostic tests, management strategies, and assessment instruments. Tables and lists of drugs are designed to facilitate appropriate prescribing. Generic and trade names are provided, as well as information on dosages, how the drugs are metabolized or excreted, and which formulations are available. Specific caveats and cautions to be observed when using the medication in older persons are also included.

The goal of *GAYF* is to reduce to a minimum the amount of time that a practicing clinician must spend searching for specific information that is needed immediately to make patient care decisions. Accordingly, the book does not attempt to explain in detail the rationale underlying the strategies presented. In many instances, these strategies have been derived from guidelines published by organizations such as the Agency for Healthcare Research and Quality, the American Geriatrics Society, the American Heart Association, and the American Diabetes Association. Many of the guidelines can be obtained from the National Guidelines Clearinghouse (http://www.guideline.gov). When no such guidelines exist, the strategies recommended herein represent the best opinions of the authors and the experts they have asked to review the chapters. In an effort to be comprehensive yet concise, references have been provided sparingly, but many others that are relevant are available from the organizations mentioned or in the most recent edition of the AGS *Geriatrics Review Syllabus*.

The authors welcome comments about the format and content of this edition of *GAYF* that may guide the preparation of future editions. All comments should be addressed to the American Geriatrics Society, Empire State Building, 350 Fifth Avenue, Suite 801, New York, NY 10118.

The authors are particularly grateful to Nancy Lundebjerg at the AGS, who has served a vital role in the development of this book and its readership. We are also grateful to the John A. Hartford Foundation for support in distributing *GAYF* to residents and medical and nurse practitioner students across the nation and for generously supporting the development of PDA versions.

We would also like to thank the following persons who have reviewed portions of the text:

Victoria Braund, MD
Catherine Dubeau, MD
Bruce A. Ferrell, MD
Perry Fine, MD
John FitzGerald, MD
Rita A. Frantz, PhD, RN
Gail Greendale, MD
Thomas Hejkel, MD
Alan Hirsh, MD
Saman Lashkari, MD
Patrick E. McBride, MD, MPH

David McCulloch, MD
Alison Moore, MD
Patricia Morrow, MS
Benoit H. Mulsant, MD
Lauren Nathan, MD
Joseph Ouslander, MD
Elizabeth Reed, MD
John Song, MD
Mary Tinetti, MD
James Webster, MD
Thomas T. Yoshikawa, MD

Guidelines of the following organizations are the basis of parts of specific chapters:

Advisory Committee on Immunization Practices
Agency for Health Care Policy and Research
  (now, Agency for Healthcare Research and Quality)
Alzheimer's Association
Amercian Academy of Neurology
American Association for Geriatric Psychiatry
American College of Cardiology
American College of Chest Physicians
American College of Gastroenterology
American College of Obstetrics and Gynecology
American College of Rheumatology
American Diabetes Association
American Geriatrics Society
American Heart Association
American Lung Association
American Pain Society
American Psychiatric Association
American Society of Anesthesiologists
American Thoracic Society
American Thyroid Association
American Urological Association
Ethnogeriatrics Committee, American Geriatrics Society
National Cholesterol Education Program
National Heart, Lung, and Blood Institute
U.S. Preventive Services Task Force
World Health Organization

The following persons have assisted the authors in planning and assembling the 2003 edition:

Managing Editor: Carol S. Goodwin
Medical Editor: Barbara B. Reitt, PhD, ELS(D), Reitt Editing Services
Medical Indexer: L. Pilar Wyman, Wyman Indexing

FORMULAS AND REFERENCE INFORMATION

Table 1. Conversions		
Temperature	**Liquid**	**Weight**
F = (1.8)C + 32	1 fl dram = 4 mL	1 lb = 0.453 kg
C = (F − 32) / (1.8)	1 fl oz = 30 mL	1 kg = 2.2 lb
	1 tsp = 5 mL	1 oz = 30 g
	1 tbsp = 15 mL	1 grain = 60 mg

FORMULAS

Alveolar-Arterial Oxygen Gradient $A - a = 148 - 1.2(Paco_2) - Pao_2$
[normal = 10 − 20 mm Hg, breathing room air at sea level]

Calculated Osmolality
2Na + glucose / 18 + BUN / 2.8 + ethanol / 4.6 + isopropanol / 6 + methanol / 3.2 +
ethylene glycol / 6.2   [normal = 280 − 295]

Golden Rules of Arterial Blood Gases
• Pco_2 change of 10 corresponds to a pH change of 0.08.
• pH change of 0.15 corresponds to base excess change of 10 mEq/L.

Creatinine Clearance
For renally eliminated drugs, dosage adjustments may be necessary if CrCl < 60.

$$\frac{IBW(140 - age)\,(0.85\,\text{if female})}{(72)\,(\text{stable creatinine})}$$

Erythrocyte Sedimentation Rate
Westergren: women = (age + 10) / 2
            men = age / 2

Ideal Body Weight
• Male = 50 kg + (2.3 kg) (each inch of height > 5 feet)
• Female = 45.5 kg + (2.3 kg) (each inch of height > 5 feet)

Lean Body Weight
IBW + 0.4 (actual body weight − IBW)

Body Mass Index

$$\frac{\text{weight in kg}}{(\text{height in meters})^2} \quad or \quad \frac{\text{weight in lb}}{(\text{height in inches})^2} \times 704.5$$

Partial Pressure of Oxygen, Arterial (Pao₂) While Breathing Room Air
100 − (age/3) estimates decline

Table 2. Motor Function by Nerve Roots			
Level	Motor Function	Level	Motor Function
C4	Spontaneous breathing	L1–L2	Hip flexion
C5	Shoulder shrug	L3	Hip adduction
C6	Elbow flexion	L4	Hip abduction
C7	Elbow extension	L5	Great toe dorsiflexion
C8/T1	Finger flexion	S1–S2	Foot plantar flexion
T1–T12	Intercostal abdominal muscles	S2–S4	Rectal tone

Table 3. Lumbosacral Nerve Root Compression			
Root	Motor	Sensory	Reflex
L4	Quadriceps	Medial foot	Knee-jerk
L5	Dorsiflexors	Dorsum of foot	Medial hamstring
S1	Plantar flexors	Lateral foot	Ankle-jerk

Figure 1. Dermatomes

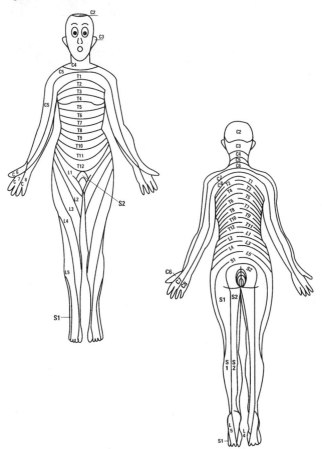

Source: *The 1999 Tarascon Pocket Pharmacopoeia.* Loma Linda, CA; Tarascon Publishing Company; 1999:7
Reprinted with permission.

ASSESSMENT AND APPROACH

ASSESSMENT

Table 4. Dimensions of Assessment*		
Domain, Dimension	**Method**	**See Page**
Medical		
Medical status	Hx, physical examination, laboratory tests	4
Medications	Medications review	9–13
Nutrition	Dietary hx	90
Dentition	Dental examination	
Mental, emotional		
Cognitive status	Mental status examination, eg, Mini-Cog, MMSE	170
Emotional status	Depression screen, eg, GDS	172–173
Spiritual status	Spiritual hx	
Physical function		
Functional status	Screen for level of function, eg, ADLs, IADLs	170–172
Balance and gait	Physical evaluation, POMA scale	174–176
Environmental		
Social, financial status	Social hx	
Environmental hazards	Home evaluation	Table 28

Note: For information on clinical uses of the domain management model, see Siebens H. Applying the domain management model in treating patients with chronic diseases. *Jt Comm J Qual Improvement* 2001;27(6):302–314.
* See Assessment Instruments, pp 170–183.

Review of Systems
Make sure to inquire about:
- Bowel patterns, especially constipation
- Cardiovascular system (eg, chest pain, SOB, claudication)
- Dizziness
- Falls
- Fatigue
- Functional change over past year or since last visit
- Hearing (see p 173) or visual changes
- Medication use (see p 9)
- Musculoskeletal stiffness or pain
- Sleep patterns
- Urinary patterns, especially incontinence
- Weight change

Physical Examination
Make sure to check:
- Height and weight
- Orthostatic BP, pulse
- Skin integrity (all surfaces)
- Vision and hearing

NURSING-HOME ASSESSMENT
Admissions Checklist
1. History, physical, labs as needed; PPD
2. Determine functional status: ADL, IADL, MSE, depression scale

3. Review medications (correlate to active diagnoses)
4. Identify medical conditions—review old records
5. Assess for presence of pain
6. Establish relationships—resident, family, staff
7. Establish advance directives
8. Formulate problem list
9. Formulate plan

Scheduled Visit Checklist
1. Evaluate patient for interval functional change
2. Check vital signs, weight, labs, consultant reports since last visit
3. Review medications (correlate to active diagnoses)
4. Sign orders
5. Address nursing staff concerns
6. Write a SOAP note (subjective data, objective data, assessment, plan)
7. Revise problem list as needed
8. Update advance directives at least yearly
9. Update resident; update family member(s) as needed

Health Maintenance
Yearly: Functional status, MSE, depression screen, vision, hearing, dental, podiatric, history, physical, creatinine, hemoglobin, other labs and preventive procedures to be decided individually
Monthly: Weight, vital signs
Ongoing: Skin integrity, pain assessment
Immunizations: influenza vaccine once/yr in the fall months; pneumococcal vaccine (*Pneumovax 23, Pnu-Immune 23*) once at age 65; consider repeat every 6–7 yr; tetanus vaccine every 10 yr

INFORMED DECISION MAKING (see also **Figure 2**)
Three elements are needed for a patient's choices to be legally, ethically valid:
• A capable decision maker: Capacity is to the decision being made; patient may be capable of making some but not all decisions. For a sufficiently impaired person, a surrogate decision maker must be involved.
• Patient's voluntary participation in the decision-making process.
• Sufficient information: Patient must be sufficiently informed; items to disclose in informed consent include:
  - Diagnosis
  - Nature, risks, costs, and benefits of possible interventions
  - Alternative treatments; relative benefits, risks, and costs
  - Likely results of no treatment
  - Likelihood of success
  - Advice or recommendation of the clinician

Figure 2. Algorithm for Informed Decision Making

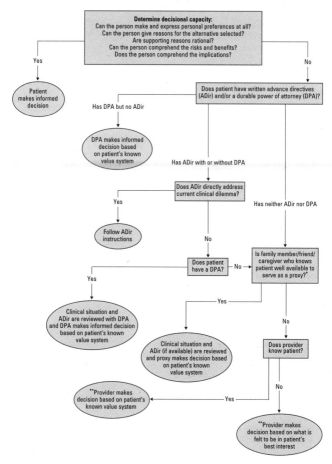

Determine decisional capacity:
Can the person make and express personal preferences at all?
Can the person give reasons for the alternative selected?
Are supporting reasons rational?
Can the person comprehend the risks and benefits?
Does the person comprehend the implications?

Yes → Patient makes informed decision

No → Does patient have written advance directives (ADir) and/or a durable power of attorney (DPA)?

Has DPA but no ADir → DPA makes informed decision based on patient's known value system

Has ADir with or without DPA → Does ADir directly address current clinical dilemma?

Yes → Follow ADir instructions

No → Does patient have a DPA?

Yes → Clinical situation and ADir are reviewed with DPA and DPA makes informed decision based on patient's known value system

No → Is family member/friend/caregiver who knows patient well available to serve as a proxy?*

Has neither ADir nor DPA → Is family member/friend/caregiver who knows patient well available to serve as a proxy?*

Yes → Clinical situation and ADir (if available) are reviewed and proxy makes decision based on patient's known value system

No → Does provider know patient?

Yes → **Provider makes decision based on patient's known value system

No → **Provider makes decision based on what is felt to be in patient's best interest

* State laws may dictate who is legal proxy
** Or court-appointed decision maker; laws vary by state

ELDER ABUSE
Risk Factors for Abuse of the Elderly Person
- Cognitive impairment
- Dependence of the abuser on the victim
- External factors causing stress
- History of violence
- Poor health and functional impairment
- Shared living arrangement
- Social isolation
- Substance abuse or mental illness on the part of the abuser

Source: Data from Lachs MS, Pillemer K. Abuse and neglect of elderly persons. *N Engl J Med.* 1995;332(7):437–443.

Presentations That Suggest Abuse or Neglect of an Elderly Patient
- Delays between an injury or illness and the seeking of medical attention
- Disparity in histories from the patient and the suspected abuser
- Implausible or vague explanations provided by either party
- Frequent visits to the emergency department for exacerbations of chronic disease despite a plan for medical care and adequate resources
- Presentation of a functionally impaired patient without his or her designated caregiver
- Laboratory findings that are inconsistent with the history provided

Source: Data from Lachs MS, Pillemer K. Abuse and neglect of elderly persons. *N Engl J Med.* 1995;332(7):437–443.

Questions To Ask About Possible Abuse
Many abuse victims can be identified simply by asking patients direct questions, eg:
- Has anyone at home ever hurt you?
- Are you afraid of anyone in your family?
- Has anyone ever scolded or threatened you?
- Are you receiving enough care at home?

Source: Jones JS. Abuse and neglect. In: Sanders AB, ed. *Emergency Care of the Elder Person.* St. Louis, MO: Beverly Cracom Publications; 1996:181. Reprinted with permission.

If Abuse Is Suspected
- Perform further evaluation, including in-depth interview (often best accomplished by Adult Protective Services staff) and careful documentation of physical and psychologic findings.
- Report suspected abuse to Adult Protective Services; 42 states have mandatory reporting laws. (See p 190 for elder abuse Web site listing the state telephone numbers.)

CROSS-CULTURAL GERIATRICS
Clinicians should remember that:
- Wide differences appear among the individuals in every ethnic group.
- Familiarity with a patient's background is useful only if his or her preferences are linked to the cultural heritage.
- Ethnic groups differ widely in
  - approach to decision making (eg, involvement of family and friends),
  - disclosure of medical information (eg, cancer diagnosis),
  - end-of-life care (eg, advance directives and resuscitation preferences).

In caring for patients of any ethnicity:
- Use the patient's preferred terminology for his or her cultural identity in conversation and in health records.
- Determine whether interpretation services are needed.
- Recognize that the patient may not conceive of illness in Western terms.
- Determine whether the patient is a refugee or survivor of violence or genocide.
- Explore early on the patient's preferences for disclosure of serious clinical findings and reconfirm at intervals.
- Ask if the patient prefers to involve or defer to others in the decision-making process.
- Follow the patient's preferences regarding gender roles.

APPROPRIATE PRESCRIBING AND PHARMACOTHERAPY

HOW TO PRESCRIBE APPROPRIATELY

- **Obtain a complete drug history.** Ask about previous treatments and responses as well as about other prescribers. Ask about allergies, OTC drugs, nutritional supplements, alternative medications, alcohol, tobacco, caffeine, and recreational drugs.
- **Avoid prescribing before a diagnosis is made.** Consider nondrug therapy. Eliminate drugs for which no diagnosis can be identified.
- **Review medications regularly and before prescribing a new medication.** D/C medications that have not had the intended response or are no longer needed. Monitor the use of prn and OTC drugs.
- **Know the actions, adverse effects, and toxicity profiles of the medications you prescribe.** Consider how these might interact or complement existing drug therapy.
- **Start chronic drug therapy at a low dose and titrate dose on the basis of tolerability and response.** Use drug levels when available.
- **Attempt to reach a therapeutic dose before switching or adding another drug.**
- **Educate patient and/or caregiver about each medication.** Include the regimen, the therapeutic goal, the cost, and potential adverse effects or drug interactions. Provide written instructions.
- **Avoid using one drug to treat the side effects of another.**
- **Attempt to use one drug to treat two or more conditions.**
- **Use combination products cautiously.** Establish need for more than one drug. Titrate individual drugs to therapeutic doses and switch to combinations if appropriate.
- **Communicate with other prescribers.** Don't assume patients will—they assume you do!
- **Avoid using drugs from the same class or with similar actions** (eg, alprazolam and zolpidem).

For more on drugs that should be avoided in all elderly patients, see p 187.

WAYS TO REDUCE MEDICATION ERRORS

- Be knowledgeable about the medication's dose, side effects, interactions, and monitoring.
- Write legibly to avoid misreading of the drug name (*Celexa* versus *Celebrex*).
- Write out the directions, strength, route, quantity, and number of refills.
- Always precede a decimal expression of <1 with a zero (0); never use a zero after a decimal.
- Avoid abbreviations, especially easily confused ones (qd and qid).
- Do not use ambiguous directions, eg, as directed (ud) or as needed.
- Include the medication's purpose in the directions (eg, for high blood pressure).
- Always re-read what you've written.

CRITERIA FOR DRUGS OF CHOICE FOR OLDER ADULTS

- Established efficacy
- Compatible safety and side-effect profile
- Low risk of drug or nutrient interactions
- Half-life <24 h with no active metabolites
- Elimination does not change with age
- Convenient dosing—single or twice daily
- Strength and dosage forms match recommended doses for older adults
- Affordable to the patient

PHARMACOLOGIC THERAPY AND AGE-ASSOCIATED CHANGES

Table 5. Age-Associated Changes in Pharmacokinetics and Pharmacodynamics			
Parameter	**Age Effect**	**Disease, Factor Effect**	**Prescribing Implications**
Absorption	Rate and extent are usually unaffected	Achlorhydria, concurrent medications, tube feedings	Drug-drug and drug-food interactions are more likely to alter absorption
Distribution	Increase in fat : water ratio. Decreased plasma protein, particularly albumin	CHF, ascites, and other conditions will increase body water	Fat-soluble drugs have a larger volume of distribution. Highly protein-bound drugs will have a greater (active) free concentration
Metabolism	Decreases in liver mass and liver blood flow may decrease drug metabolism	Smoking, genotype, concurrent drug therapy, alcohol and caffeine intake may have more effect than aging	Lower doses may be therapeutic
Elimination	Primarily renal. Age-related decrease in GFR	Renal impairment with acute and chronic diseases; decreased muscle mass results in lower creatinine production	Serum creatinine not a reliable measure of renal function; best to estimate CrCl using formula on p 1
Pharmaco-dynamics	Less predictable and often altered drug response at usual or lower concentrations	Drug-drug and drug-disease interactions may alter responses	Prolonged pain relief with morphine at lower doses. Increased sedation and postural instability to benzodiazepines. Altered sensitivity to β-blockers

AGGRAVATING FACTORS

Drug-Food or -Nutrient Interactions

Physical Interactions: Mg^{++}, Ca^{++}, Fe^{++}, Al^{++}, or zinc can lower oral absorption of quinolone antibiotics, and tube feedings will decrease absorption of oral phenytoin and levothyroxine.

Decreased Drug Effect: Warfarin and vitamin K-containing foods (eg, green leafy vegetables, broccoli, brussels sprouts, greens, cabbage).

Decreased Oral Intake or Appetite: Drugs can alter the taste of food (dysgeusia) or decrease saliva production (xerostomia), making mastication and swallowing difficult. Drugs associated with dysgeusia include captopril and clarithromycin. Drugs that can cause xerostomia include antihistamines, antidepressants, antipsychotics, clonidine, and diuretics.

Drug-Drug Interactions

A drug's effect can be increased or decreased by another drug because of impaired absorption (eg, sucralfate and ciprofloxacin), displacement from protein-binding sites (eg, warfarin and sulfonamides), inhibition or induction of metabolic enzymes (see **Table 6**), or because two or more drugs have a similar pharmacologic effect (eg, potassium-sparing diuretics, potassium supplements, and ACE inhibitors).

Digoxin: Digoxin levels must be monitored with concomitant administration of many other drugs.

The following **increase** digoxin concentration or effect, or both:

amiodarone	hydroxychloroquine	quinine
diltiazem	ibuprofen	spironolactone
erythromycin	indomethacin	tetracycline
esmolol	nifedipine	tolbutamide
flecainide	quinidine	verapamil

The following **decrease** digoxin concentration or effect, or both:

aminosalicylic acid	colestipol	sulfasalazine
antacids	kaolin pectin	St. John's wort
antineoplastics	metoclopramide	
cholestyramine	psyllium	

Enzyme Inhibitors and Inducers: **Table 6** is a list of common drug-drug interactions via this mechanism.

Table 6. Selected CYP Isozyme Substrates, Inducers, and Inhibitors

Substrates*		Isozyme	Inducers**	Inhibitors†
APAP Clozapine Desipramine Estradiol Imipramine	Nortriptyline Olanzapine Warfarin	CYP1A2	Carbamazepine Cigarette smoke Omeprazole Phenobarbital Phenytoin Rifampin	Amiodarone Cimetidine Diltiazem Estradiol Fluoroquinolones Fluvoxamine Isoniazid Ketoconazole
Celecoxib Fluvastatin Phenytoin Warfarin		CYP2C9	Carbamazepine Phenobarbital Phenytoin Rifampin	Amiodarone Cimetidine Fluconazole Fluvoxamine Isoniazid Omeprazole Propoxyphene Valproic acid
Codeine‡ Dextromethorphan Haloperidol Metoprolol Most TCAs	Paroxetine Risperidone Timolol Tramadol‡ Venlafaxine	CYP2D6		Amiodarone Bupropion Celecoxib Cimetidine Diltiazem Fluoxetine Paroxetine Propoxyphene Quinidine Valproic acid

Alprazolam
Amiodarone
Atorvastatin
Buspirone
Carbamazepine
Clarithromycin
Clozapine
Codeine
Cyclosporine
Dihydropyridine
  calcium channel
  blockers
Diltiazem
Erythromycin
Estradiol
Fluoxetine
Haloperidol
Itraconazole
Ketoconazole
	Lovastatin
	Nefazodone
	Omeprazole
	Pioglitazone
	Quetiapine
	Risperidone
	Sildenafil
	Simvastatin
	Triazolam
	Venlafaxine
	Verapamil
	Warfarin
	Ziprasidone
	Zolpidem
		CYP3A4	Carbamazepine
			Glucocorticoids
			Griseofulvin
			Oxcarbazepine
			Phenobarbital
			Phenytoin
			Pioglitazone
			Rifabutin
			Rifampin
			St. John's wort
				Amiodarone
				Cimetidine
				Clarithromycin
				Cyclosporine
				Diltiazem
				Erythromycin
				Fluconazole
				Fluoxetine
				Fluvoxamine
				Grapefruit juice
				Haloperidol
				Isoniazid
				Itraconazole
				Ketoconazole
				Propoxyphene
				Nefazodone
				Quinidine
				Sertraline
				Verapamil

* Substrate: a drug metabolized by the isozyme.
** Inducer: a drug that increases the capacity of the isozyme to metabolize the substrate and potentially decreases the therapeutic effect of the substrate.
† Inhibitor: a drug that prevents the isozyme from metabolizing the substrate and increases the risk for toxicity or therapeutic failure of the substrate.
‡ Analgesic effect decreased because of inhibition of substrate metabolism to its active metabolite by an inhibitor.
Note: The list of medications is not comprehensive, but represents medications often prescribed for older patients or medications involved in very serious drug interactions (eg, cyclosporine). Some interactions have in vivo or in vitro documentation, whereas others are theoretical. For more information, consult a drug-drug interaction text or Internet resource, eg, http://medicine.iupui.edu/flockhart/.

APPROPRIATE PRESCRIBING

Drug-Disease Interactions

Table 7. Drug-Disease Interactions		
Disease	**Drugs**	**Adverse Effects**
Benign prostatic hyperplasia	Anticholinergics, calcium channel blockers, decongestants	Urinary retention
Cardiac conduction abnormalities	Verapamil, TCAs, β-blockers (all routes)	Heart block
Asthma	β-blockers (all routes), narcotic analgesics	Bronchoconstriction, respiratory depression
Chronic renal insufficiency	NSAIDs, contrast agents, aminoglycosides	Acute renal failure
Dementia	Anticholinergics, benzodiazepines, opiates, TCAs, antiparkinsonian agents	Delirium
Diabetes mellitus	Diuretics, corticosteroids	Hyperglycemia
Angle-closure glaucoma	Anticholinergics	Acute ↑ in IOP
Hypertension	NSAIDs	Increased BP
Hypokalemia	Digoxin	Cardiac arrhythmias
Hyponatremia	Oral hypoglycemics, diuretics, SSRIs, carbamazepine, antipsychotics	↓ Serum sodium
Peptic ulcer	NSAIDs	Upper GI bleeding
Postural hypotension	Diuretics, TCAs, MAOIs, vasodilators, antiparkinsonian agents	Syncope, falls, hip fracture

Source: Adapted from Parker BM, Cusack BJ. Pharmacology and appropriate prescribing. In: Reuben DB, Yoshikawa TT, Besdine RW, eds. *Geriatrics Review Syllabus: A Core Curriculum in Geriatric Medicine.* 3rd ed. Dubuque, Iowa: Kendall/Hunt Publishing Company for the American Geriatrics Society; 1996:33. Reprinted with permission.

ALCOHOL AND TOBACCO ABUSE

ALCOHOL ABUSE
Definition
Possible Alcohol Dependence—DSM-IV: Three or more of the following:
- Tolerance, requiring more alcohol to get "high"
- Withdrawal, or drinking to relieve, prevent withdrawal
- Drinking in larger amounts, or for a longer time than intended
- Persistent desire to drink, or unsuccessful efforts to control drinking
- Spending a lot of time obtaining, using alcohol, or recovering from effects
- Giving up important occupational, social, or recreational activities because of drinking
- Drinking despite persistent or recurrent physical or psychologic problems caused or worsened by alcohol

Possible Alcohol Abuse—DSM-IV: Recurring problems with one or more of the following:
- Drinking resulting in the failure to fulfill major obligations at work or in the home
- Drinking in situations where it is physically hazardous
- Alcohol-related legal problems
- Continued drinking despite social problems caused or worsened by alcohol

Hazardous Drinking: WHO definition—use of alcohol that places a person at risk of physical or psychologic complications. Increases risk of HTN, some cancers (eg, head and neck, esophagus, breast in women), and cirrhosis (higher in women). Possible increased risk for hip fracture and other injury.

Evaluation
Alcohol dependence or abuse is often missed in older persons because of reduced social and occupational functioning; signs more often are poor self-care, malnutrition, and medical illness.

Alcohol Misuse Screening: CAGE questionnaire has been validated in the older population.

C Have you ever felt you should **C**ut down?
A Does others' criticism of your drinking **A**nnoy you?
G Have you ever felt **G**uilty about drinking?
E Have you ever had an "**E**ye opener" to steady your nerves or get rid of a hangover?
 (*Positive response to any suggests problem drinking.*)

Detecting Harmful Drinking (≥ *2 drinks/d for women,* ≥ *3 drinks/d for men is potentially harmful*): May be missed by CAGE; ask
- How many days per week?
- How many drinks on those days?
- Maximum intake on any one day?

- What type (ie, beer, wine, or liquor)?
- What is in "a drink"?

Aggravating Factors
Alcohol and Aging: Higher blood levels per amount consumed due to decreased lean body mass and total body water; concomitant medications may interact with alcohol.
Age-related Diseases: Cognitive impairment, HTN.
Medications: Many drug interactions, eg, APAP, antihypertensives, NSAIDs, sedatives, antidepressants.

Management
Alcohol Guidelines for Moderate Drinking: No more than 1 drink/d after age 65; 1 drink/d probably reduces cardiovascular risk.
Psychosocial Interventions:
• Problem drinking or alcohol misuse: Brief intervention; educate patient on effects of current drinking, point out current adverse effects.
• Alcohol dependence or abuse: Self-help groups (eg, Alcoholics Anonymous); professional (eg, psychodynamic, cognitive-behavioral, counseling, social support, family therapy, age-specific inpatient or outpatient).
• Drug therapy: Naltrexone *(Depade, reVia, Trexan)* 25 mg × 2d, then 50 mg qd [T: 50]. Monitor liver enzymes; useful adjunct to psychosocial therapy; contraindicated in renal failure; ~10% get nausea, headache (L, K).
• Acute alcohol withdrawal: See p 40.

SMOKING CESSATION

Table 8. Pharmacotherapy for Tobacco Abuse			
Drug	**Dosage**	**Formulations**	**Comment (Metabolism, Excretion)**
Tobacco Abuse			
Bupropion* (*Wellbutrin SR, Zyban*)	150 mg bid × 7–12 wk	[SR: 100, 150]	Combined with nicotine replacement, doubles quit rate to 30% at 12 mo; contraindicated with seizure disorders (L)
Nicotine Replacement**			
Transdermal patches† (eg, *Habitrol, Nicoderm*)	21 mg/d × 4–8 wk 14 mg/d × 2–4 wk 7 mg/d × 2–4 wk	[7, 14, 21]	Apply to clean, nonhairy skin on upper torso, rotate sites; start 14 mg/d with cardiovascular disease or body wt < 100 lb or if smoking < 10 cigarettes/d (L)
(*Nicotrol*)	15 mg/d × 8 wk 10 mg/d × 4–6 wk 5 mg/d × 4–6 wk	[5, 10, 15]	Gradually released over 16 h (L)
(*ProStep*)	22 mg/d × 4–8 wk 11 mg/d × 4–8 wk	[11, 22]	Persons < 100 lb start lower dose; reduce or D/C after 4–8 wk (L)
Polacrilex gum (*Nicorette*)	9–12 pieces/d	[2, 4]	Chew 1 piece when urge to smoke; usual 10–12 d, maximum 30/d; 4 mg for smokers > 21 cigarettes/d (L)

(continues)

Table 8. Pharmacotherapy for Tobacco Abuse (cont.)			
Drug	Dosage	Formulations	Comment (Metabolism, Excretion)
Nasal spray (*Nicotrol NS*)	1 spr each nostril q 30–60 min	[0.5 mg/spr]	Do not exceed 5 applications/h or 40 in 24 h (L)
Inhaler[††] (*Nicotrol Inhaler*)	6–16 cartridges/d	[4 mg delivered/cartridge]	Maximum 16 cartridges/d with gradual reduction after 6–12 wk if needed (L)

* Bupropion is FDA approved. Nortriptyline is an effective alternative. Hughes JR, Stead LF, Lancaster T. Antidepressants for smoking cessation. *Cochrano Database Syst Rev* 2002; 1:000031.

** Best used in combination with smoking cessation program; dyspepsia is most common drug-related side effect.

† In patients receiving > 600 mg cimetidine, reduce to next lower patch dose.

†† Available by prescription only.

WARFARIN THERAPY
Prescribing Warfarin
- Initiate therapy by giving warfarin (*Coumadin, Carfin, Sofarin*) 2–5 mg/d as fixed dose [T: 1, 2, 2.5, 3, 4, 5, 6, 7.5, 10]; reduce dose if INR > 2.5 on day 3.
- Half-life is 31–51 h; steady state is achieved on day 5–7 of fixed dose.
- The following drugs **increase** INR in conjunction with warfarin:

alcohol use (binge)	ASA (> 3 g/d)	SSRIs
allopurinol	corticosteroids	tamoxifen
amiodarone	NSAIDs	vitamin E (≥ 400 IU)
antibiotics	omeprazole	
APAP (> 1.3 g/d >1 wk;	phenytoin	
monitor INR)	propoxyphene	

- The following drugs **decrease** INR in conjunction with warfarin:

alcohol use (moderate)	cholestyramine	sucralfate
barbiturates	estrogens	vitamin K
carbamazepine	rifampin	

Table 9. Anticoagulation Indicated in the Absence of Active Bleeding or Severe Bleeding Risk		
Condition	**Target INR**	**Duration of Therapy**
Hip or major knee surgery	2.0–3.0	7–10 days or until patient is ambulatory
Isolated symptomatic calf vein thrombosis	2.0–3.0	At least 3 mo
Initial idiopathic vein thrombosis	2.0–3.0	At least 6 mo
PE	2.0–3.0	6 mo
Recurrent thromboses or PE	2.0–3.0	At least 12 mo
Atrial fibrillation	2.0–3.0	Indefinitely
Mitral valvular heart disease with hx of systemic embolization or left atrial diameter > 5.5 cm	2.0–3.0	Indefinitely
Cardiomyopathy with EF < 25%	2.0–3.0	Indefinitely
Mechanical mitral heart valve	2.5–3.5	Indefinitely
Mechanical aortic heart valve	2.0–3.0	Indefinitely
Prosthetic heart valve	2.0–3.0	3 mo
Acute MI complicated by severe LV dysfunction, CHF, previous emboli, mural thrombus on echocardiography	2.0–3.0	1–3 mo

Cessation of Anticoagulation Prior to Surgery
- If INR is between 2.0 and 3.0, hold warfarin 4 doses prior to surgery; longer if INR > 3.0.
- If patient has a mechanical valve, heparin should be used after warfarin is held prior to surgery.

Table 10. Treatment of Warfarin Overdose		
INR	**Clinical Situation**	**Action**
≥ 3.5 and < 5.0	No significant bleeding	Omit next warfarin dose and/or lower dose
≥ 5.0 and < 9.0	No significant bleeding	Omit next 1–2 doses of warfarin and restart therapy at lower dose; alternatively, omit 1 dose and give vitamin K (VK) 1.0–2.5 mg po
≥ 9.0	No significant bleeding	D/C warfarin and give VK 3.0–5.0 mg po; give additional VK orally if INR is not substantially reduced in 24–48 h. Restart warfarin at lower dose when INR is therapeutic.
≥ 3.0 and < 20.0	Serious bleeding	D/C warfarin; give VK 1.0–10.0 mg by slow IV infusion, supplemented with fresh frozen plasma or prothrombin complex concentrate depending on urgency of situation; check INR q 6h; repeat VK q 12h as needed
Any elevation	Life-threatening bleeding	D/C warfarin; give VK 10.0 mg by slow IV infusion, supplemented with prothrombin complex concentrate; repeat this treatment as needed

Source: Data from American College of Chest Physicians Consensus Panel on Antithrombotic Therapy. Ansell J, Dalen J, Anderson D, et al. Managing oral anticoagulant therapy. In: Sixth ACCP Consensus Conference on Antithrombotic Therapy. *Chest.* 2001; 119(1 Suppl):22S–38S.

ACUTE ANTICOAGULATION

Table 11. Weight-Based Heparin Dosage	
Initial	80 U/kg bolus = _____ U (not to exceed 10,000 U) 18 U/kg/h = _____ U/h (not to exceed 1500 U)
PTT < 35	80 U/kg bolus = _____ U Increase drip 4 U/kg/h = _____ U/h
PTT 35 to 45	40 U/kg bolus = _____ U Increase drip 2 U/kg/h = _____ U/h
PTT 46 to 70	No change
PTT 71 to 90	Reduce drip to 2 U/kg/h = _____ U/h Hold heparin for 1 h Reduce drip 3 U/kg/h = _____ U/h

Note: Order PTT 6 h after any dosage change, adjusting heparin infusion by the sliding scale until PTT is therapeutic (46–70 sec). When two consecutive PTTs are therapeutic, order PTT (and readjust heparin drip as needed) q 24 h.
Source: Adapted from Figure 3 in Raschke RA, Reilly BM, Guidry JR, et al. Weight-based heparin dosing nomogram compared with a standard care nomogram. *Ann Intern Med.* 1993;119(9):874. Reprinted with permission.

Table 12. Other Anticoagulants				
Class, Agent	Prophylaxis Dosing by Indication*	Treatment Dosing by Indication	Half-Life	Comments (Metabolism, Excretion)
LMWH				
Enoxaparin (*Lovenox*)	Elective hip or knee replacement: 30 mg SC bid or 0.5 mg/kg SC q 12 h if > 64 yr or < 45 kg; High-risk elective hip replacement or surgery: 40 mg SC qd	DVT or PE or acute coronary syndrome**: 1 mg/kg SC q 12 h; Inpatient treatment for DVT with or without PE or outpatient treatment for DVT without PE: 1.5 mg/kg SC qd	3–6 h	Bleeding, anemia, hyperkalemia, hyper-transaminasemia, thrombocytopenia, thrombocytosis, urticaria, angioedema (K)
Dalteparin (*Fragmin*)	DVT: Hip fracture surgery: 2500 or 5000 U SC pre-op, then 5000 U SC qd; Abdominal surgery: DVT risk high: 5000 U SC pre-op, then qd ×5–10 d	DVT: 100 U/kg SC bid or 200 U/kg SC qd; Unstable angina, non-Q-wave MI: 120 U/kg SC q 12 h × 5–8 d. Max 10,000 U	3–4 h	Same (K)
Tinzaparin (*Innohep*)	NA	DVT or PE: 175 anti-Xa IU/kg SC qd	3–4 h	Same (K)
Heparinoid				
Danaparoid (*Orgaran*)	Elective hip replacement: 750 U SC q 12 h begun 1–4 h post-op or 2 or more h post-op	DVT or PE: initial weight-based dose IV; < 55 kg: 1250 anti-Xa U; 55–90 kg: 2500 anti-Xa U; > 90 kg: 3750 anti-Xa U; All are followed with 400 U/h × 4 h, then 300 U/h × 4 h, then 150-200 U/h maintenance dose; If DVT or PE > 5 d old: < 90 kg: 1250 U IV, then 750 U SC qd × 3 d; > 90 kg: 1250 U IV, then 1250 U SC qd × 3 d	24 h	Same, fever (22%), approved for DVT prophylaxis in total hip replacement surgery (K)

(*continues*)

Table 12. Other Anticoagulants (cont.)				
Class, Agent	Prophylaxis Dosing by Indication*	Treatment Dosing by Indication	Half-Life	Comments (Metabolism, Excretion)
Factor Xa Inhibitor				
Fondaparinux (*Arixtra*)	Hip fracture surgery or elective hip or knee replacement: ≥ 50 kg: 2.5 mg SC qd, starting 6–8 h post-op for up to 11 d	NA	17–21	Not for use in patients < 50 kg or CrCl < 30 mL/min. Use with caution in patients > 75 yr because of ↑ risk of bleeding
Thombolytics				
Streptokinase (*Kabiki-nase, Streptase*)	NA	Acute MI: 1.5 million U IV over 60 min Acute PE: 250,000 U IV over 30 min, then 100,000 U/h for 24 h	1.3 h	Risk of hemorrhage ↑ with age and higher BMI; HTN, hallucination, agitation, confusion, serum sickness (L)

*According to the American College of Chest Physicians guidelines, all patients over the age of 60 are considered high risk for general surgery.
**Prevention of ischemic complications with unstable angina or non-Q-wave MI.

ANXIETY

DIAGNOSIS

Anxiety disorders are less prevalent in elderly than in younger adults. New-onset anxiety in elderly persons is often secondary to physical illness, depression, medication side effects, or withdrawal from drugs.

DSM-IV recognizes several anxiety disorders:
(***Bold*** *type indicates the most common anxiety disorders occurring in older persons.*)
- Acute stress disorder
- Agoraphobia without a history of panic
- **GAD**
- **Anxiety disorder due to a general medical condition**
- Obsessive-compulsive disorder (OCD)
- Panic disorder, with or without agoraphobia
- Post-traumatic stress disorder
- Social phobia
- Specific phobia
- Substance-induced anxiety disorder

DSM-IV Criteria for GAD
- Excessive anxiety and worry on more days than not for ≥ 6 mo, about a number of events or activities
- Difficulty controlling the worry
- Anxiety and worry associated with ≥ 3 of 6 symptoms:
  - restlessness or feeling keyed up or on edge
  - being easily fatigued
  - difficulty concentrating or mind going blank
  - irritability
  - muscle tension
  - sleep disturbance (difficulty falling or staying asleep, or restless unsatisfying sleep)
- Focus of anxiety and worry not confined to features of an Axis I disorder (primary psychiatric disorder); often, about routine life circumstances; may shift from one concern to another
- Anxiety, worry, or physical symptoms cause clinically significant distress or impairment in social, occupational, or other important areas of functioning
- Disturbance not due to the direct physiologic effects of a drug of abuse or a medication or to a medical condition; does not occur exclusively during a mood disorder, psychotic disorder, or a pervasive development disorder.

DSM-IV Criteria for Panic Attack
Discrete period of intense fear or discomfort with $\geq$ 4 of the following (also, must peak within 10 min):

- Palpitations, rapid HR
- Sweating
- Trembling or shaking
- Sensations of SOB or smothering
- Choking feeling
- Chest pain or discomfort
- Nausea or abdominal distress
- Feeling dizzy, unsteady, lightheaded, or faint
- Feelings of unreality or being detached from self
- Fear of losing control or going crazy
- Fear of dying
- Paresthesias
- Chills or hot flushes

Differential Diagnosis
- Physical conditions producing anxiety
  - Cardiovascular: Arrhythmias, angina, MI, CHF
  - Endocrine: Hyperthyroidism, hypoglycemia, pheochromocytoma
  - Neurologic: Movement disorders, temporal lobe epilepsy, AD, stroke
  - Respiratory: COPD, asthma, pulmonary embolism
- Medications producing anxiety
  - Caffeine
  - Corticosteroids
  - Nicotine
  - Psychotropics: Antidepressants, antipsychotics, stimulants
  - Sympathomimetics: Pseudoephedrine, β-agonists
  - Thyroid hormones: Overreplacement
- Withdrawal states: alcohol, sedatives, hypnotics, benzodiazepines
- Depression

EVALUATION
- Past psychiatric hx
- Drug review: Prescribed, OTC, alcohol, caffeine
- Mental status evaluation
- Physical examination: Focus on signs and symptoms of anxiety (eg, tachycardia, hyperpnea, sweating, tremor)
- Laboratory tests: Consider CBC, blood glucose, TSH, B_{12}, ECG, oxygen saturation, drug and alcohol screening

MANAGEMENT
Nonpharmacologic
Cognitive-behavior therapy may be useful for GAD, panic disorder, and OCD.
May be effective alone but mostly used in conjunction with pharmacotherapy.
Requires a cognitively intact, motivated patient.

Pharmacologic
Antidepressants Approved for Anxiety Disorders: See **Table 22** for dosing.
- Obsessive-compulsive: fluoxetine, fluvoxamine, paroxetine, sertraline; secondary choices include β-blockers and atypical antipsychotics
- Panic: sertraline, paroxetine; secondary choices include β-blockers and atypical antipsychotics
- Social phobia: paroxetine

ANXIETY

- Generalized anxiety: venlafaxine, paroxetine
- Post-traumatic stress: paroxetine, sertraline

Buspirone (BuSpar):
- Serotonin 1A partial agonist effective in GAD and anxiety symptoms accompanying general medical illness
- Not effective for acute anxiety, panic, or OCD
- May take 2–4 wk for therapeutic response
- Recommended geriatric dosage: 15–20 mg bid [T: 5, 7.5, 10, 15, 30]
- No dependence, tolerance, withdrawal, CNS depression, or significant drug-drug interactions

Benzodiazepines:
- Most often used for acute anxiety, GAD, panic, OCD
- Preferred: Intermediate–half-life drugs inactivated by direct conjugation in liver and therefore less affected by aging

Table 13. Benzodiazepines for Anxiety Recommended for Geriatric Patients		
Drug	Dosage	Formulations
Lorazepam (*Ativan*)	0.5–2 mg in 2–3 divided doses	[T: 0.5, 1, 2; S: 2 mg/mL; Inj: 2 mg/mL]
Oxazepam (*Serax*)	10–15 mg bid–tid	[T: 10, 15, 30]

- Long-acting benzodiazepines (eg, flurazepam, diazepam, chlordiazepoxide): Linked to cognitive impairment, falls, sedation, psychomotor impairment
- Problems: Dependence, tolerance, withdrawal, more so with short-acting benzodiazepines; seizure risk with alprazolam withdrawal
- Potentially fatal if combined with alcohol or other CNS depressants
- Only short-term (60–90 d) use recommended

DIAGNOSTIC CARDIAC TESTS

Angina, Coronary Artery Disease
- Cardiac catheterization is the gold standard.
- Stress testing: The heart is stressed either through exercise (treadmill, stationary bicycle) or, if the patient cannot exercise or the ECG is markedly abnormal, with pharmacologic agents (dipyridamole, adenosine, dobutamine). Exercise stress tests can be performed with or without cardiac imaging, while pharmacologic stress tests always include imaging. Imaging can be accomplished by a nuclear isotope (eg, thallium) or echocardiography.
- Cardiac enzymes if acute chest pain (troponin, CPK)
- Electron-beam computed tomography (EBCT) is not currently recommended as a screening test for CAD.

Congestive Heart Failure
- First line: ECG, CXR, echocardiogram (provides valuable information about left ventricular size and function, valvular function; difficult to perform in patients with obesity or lung disease)
- Measurement of plasma brain natriuretic peptide (BNP) can be helpful in diagnosing acute heart failure. A BNP > 100 pg/mL strongly suggests decreased LV function or acute CHF.
- Other: Radionuclide ventriculography, which measures EF more precisely, provides a better evaluation of right ventricular function, and is more expensive than echocardiography

Palpitations, Presyncope, Syncope
- First line: CXR, ECG, 24- or 48-h rhythm (Holter) monitoring
- Other: Ambulatory BP monitoring, tilt-table testing, electrophysiological studies, implantable cardiac monitors

ACUTE MYOCARDIAL INFARCTION

Evaluation and Assessment
- Presentation frequently atypical—suspect MI with atypical chest pain; arm, jaw, or abdominal pain (with or without nausea); acute functional decline.
- As in younger persons, diagnosis is made by cardiac enzyme rises, with or without ECG changes. Serial enzyme measurements are necessary to exclude MI.
  - Both creatine kinase MB isoenzymes (CK-MB) and cardiac troponins T and I usually become elevated 4 h following myocardial injury.
  - CK-MB subforms are the most sensitive and specific test for detecting MI in the first 6 h, but troponin remains elevated longer.
  - Elevated troponin in the face of normal CK-MB can indicate increased risk of MI in the ensuing 6 mo.
  - Troponins are not useful for detecting reinfarction within 1st wk of an MI. CK-MB is the preferred marker for early reinfarction.

- Both CK-MB and cardiac troponins can exhibit false-positive results that are due to subclinical ischemic myocardial injury or nonischemic myocardial injury.
• Risk factors for acute MI in older adults:

Strong:
- Previous MI or angina
- Age
- Diabetes mellitus
- Hypertension
- Smoking
- Severe coronary artery calcification

Weak:
- Dyslipidemia (except in those with overt coronary disease)
- Family hx
- Obesity
- Sedentary life style

Management
Thrombolytic Therapy for Q-wave MI (Chest Pain < 12 h, ≥ 1 mm ST-Segment Elevation):
• Age is not a contraindication.
• Absolute contraindications (ACC/AHA):
  - Prior hemorrhagic stroke
  - Other stroke or intracerebral event in past yr
  - Active internal bleeding
  - Known intracranial neoplasm
  - Aortic dissection
• Relative contraindications:
  - BP > 180/110 on presentation
  - Hx of prior stroke or known intracerebral pathology not covered in absolute contraindications
  - Current therapeutic INR ≥ 3
  - Known bleeding diathesis
  - Recent (< 3 wk) major surgery
  - Prolonged (> 10 min) or traumatic CPR
  - Recent (< 2–4 wk) trauma or internal bleeding
  - Noncompressible vascular puncture
  - Active peptic ulcer
  - Hx of severe, chronic HTN
  - For streptokinase or anistreplase, prior exposure (5 d–2 yr) or prior allergic reactions

Surgery:
Percutaneous transluminal coronary angioplasty (PTCA), preferably with stent placement, or emergent coronary artery bypass grafting (CABG) are alternatives to thrombolytic therapy.

Acute Pharmacologic Management (give at initial presentation):
For both Q-wave MI and acute coronary syndrome (unstable angina or non-Q-wave MI)
• ASA, at least 160 mg qd initially, should be started at the time of MI and continued indefinitely at 81–325 mg/d.
• In addition to ASA therapy, clopidogrel (*Plavix*) 300 mg po initially followed by 75 mg po qd [T:75] can lower risk of recurrent MI; combination therapy with ASA and clopidogrel is also associated with higher bleeding complications, so therapy should be considered only for those at low bleeding risk.
• Heparin should be given acutely. For patients undergoing thrombolytic therapy or immediate PTCA, those with continuing pain or those with indications for warfarin therapy (see p 26), give 5000 units bolus IV + 1000 units/h IV; check activated PTT q 6 h (target 1.5–2.0 × control). Otherwise, give LMWH (eg, enoxaparin [*Lovenox*]) 1 mg/kg SC q 12 h until patient is fully ambulatory.

- If PTCA is expected within 24 h, IV antiplatelet therapy is also indicated with a glycoprotein IIb/IIIa inhibitor (eg, abciximab [*ReoPro*] 0.25 mg/kg IV bolus followed by IV infusion of 0.125 μg/kg/min [max 10 μg/min] *or* eptifibatide [*Integrilin*] 180 μg/kg IV bolus [max 22.6 mg] followed by 2 μg/kg max up to 15 mg/h *or* tirofiban [*Aggrastat*] 0.4 μg/kg/min × 30 min, then 0.1 μg/kg/min).
- β-Blockers should be given acutely and continued chronically unless systolic failure or pronounced bradycardia is present. Acute phase: Atenolol (*Tenormin*), 5 mg IV over 5 min and repeat in 10 min; or metoprolol (*Lopressor*) 5 mg IV q 5 min up to a total of 15 mg. Begin chronic phase within 1–2 h: atenolol 25–100 mg po qd or metoprolol, 50–200 mg po bid.
- Nitroglycerin is indicated acutely for persistent ischemia, hypertension, large anterior infarction, or CHF. Begin at 5–10 μg/min IV and titrate to pain relief, SBP > 90, or resolution of ECG abnormalities.
- Oxygen: 2–4 L/min via nasal cannula should be given acutely.

Subacute Pharmacologic Management (give during hospitalization): For both Q-wave MI and acute coronary syndrome (unstable angina or non-Q-wave MI)
- Patients with hematocrit ≤ 30 and who are not in CHF should be transfused to achieve hematocrit > 33.
- ACE inhibitors should be started within 1st 24 h following MI with ST-segment elevation, particularly in cases with systolic dysfunction, eg: captopril (*Capoten*), 6.25–25 mg po bid–tid; enalapril (*Vasotec*), 2.5–20 mg po qd/bid; lisinopril (*Prinivil, Zestril*), 2.5–20 mg po qd. Start at low dose and titrate to maximum tolerated dose.
- Warfarin therapy is indicated in post-MI patients with atrial fibrillation, left ventricular thrombosis, or large anterior infarction (see **Table 9**).
- Lipid-lowering therapy (see Dyslipidemia section, p 28) to achieve target levels (total cholesterol < 160 mg/dL, LDL cholesterol < 100 mg/dL, HDL cholesterol > 45 mg/dL) should be initiated by the time of hospital discharge.
- At time of discharge, prescribe rapid-acting nitrates prn: Sublingual nitroglycerin or nitroglycerin spray every 5 min for maximum of 3 doses in 15 min. See **Table 14**.
- Longer-acting nitrates should be prescribed if symptomatic angina and treatment will be medical rather than surgical or angioplasty. May be combined with β-blockers or calcium channel blockers, or both. See **Table 14**.
- Calcium channel blockers should be used cautiously for management of angina only in non-Q-wave infarctions without systolic dysfunction and a contraindication to β-blockers.

Table 14. Nitrate Dosages and Formulations		
Drug	**Dosage**	**Formulations**
Oral		
Isosorbide dinitrate (*Isordil, Sorbitrate*)	10–40 mg tid (6 h apart)	[T: 5, 10, 20, 30, 40; CT: 5, 10]
Isosorbide dinitrate SR (*Isordil Tembids, Dilatrate SR*)	40–80 mg bid–tid	[T: 40]
Isosorbide mononitrate (*ISMO, Monoket*)	20 mg bid (8 AM and 3 PM)	[T: 10, 20]
Isosorbide mononitrate SR (*Imdur*)	start 30–60 mg qd; max 240 mg/d	[T: 30, 60, 120]
Nitroglycerin (*Nitro-Bid*)	2.5–9 mg bid–tid	[T: 2.5, 6.5, 9]

CARDIOVASCULAR

Table 14. Nitrate Dosages and Formulations (cont.)		
Drug	Dosage	Formulations
Sublingual		
Isosorbide dinitrate (*Isordil, Sorbitrate*)	1 tablet prn	[T: 2.5, 5, 10]
Nitroglycerin (*Nitrostat*)	0.4 mg prn	[T: 0.15, 0.3, 0.4, 0.6]
Oral spray		
Nitroglycerin (*Nitrolingual*)	1–2 spr prn; max 3/15 min	[0.4 mg/spr]
Ointment		
Nitroglycerin 2% (*Nitro-Bid, Nitrol*)	start 0.5–4 inches q 4–8 h	[2%]
Transdermal		
Nitroglycerin (*Deponit*)	1 pat 12–14 h/d	[0.2, 0.4 (mg/h)]
(*Minitran*)		[0.1, 0.2, 0.4, 0.6]
(*Nitrek*)		[0.2, 0.4, 0.6 (mg/h)]
(*Nitro-Our*)		[0.1, 0.2, 0.3, 0.4, 0.6, 0.8]
(*Nitrodisc*)		[0.2, 0.3, 0.4]
(*Transderm-Nitro*)		[0.1, 0.2, 0.4, 0.6, 0.8]

CONGESTIVE HEART FAILURE
Evaluation and Assessment
- All patients initially presenting with CHF should have an echocardiogram to evaluate left ventricular function. An ejection fraction (EF) of < 40% indicates systolic dysfunction. Heart failure with an EF ≥ 40% indicates diastolic dysfunction.
- Other routine assessment tests: ECG, CXR, CBC, electrolytes, creatinine, albumin, LFTs, TSH, UA
- New York Heart Association (NYHA) classification of cardiac disability:
  - Class I—cardiac disease without resulting limitation of physical activity
  - Class II—comfortable at rest, but symptoms (dyspnea, fatigue, palpitation, angina) on normal physical activity
  - Class III—comfortable at rest, but symptoms on slight physical activity
  - Class IV—symptoms at rest

Management*
Nonpharmacologic:
- Exercise: Regular walking or cycling for NYHA Class I–III disability
- Measure weight daily
- Salt restriction: 3 g sodium diet is reasonable goal; 2 g in severe CHF

Pharmacologic: For information on drug dosages and side effects not listed below, see **Table 16**. Clinicians should be aware that efficacy of different medications may vary significantly across racial and ethnic groups; eg, blacks may require higher doses of ACE inhibitors and β-blockers.
- Systolic dysfunction:
  - Diuretics if volume overload
  - ACE inhibitors to target levels, eg, 150 mg/d of captopril or ≥ 20 mg/d of enalapril or lisinopril

- For all stable patients with little or no fluid retention, a β-blocker (metoprolol XL [*Toprol-XL*] 12.5–25 mg po qd initially, maximum 200 mg/d; or bisoprolol [*Zebeta*] 1.25 mg po qd initially, maximum 5 mg qd); or carvedilol (*Coreg*) 3.125 mg po bid initially, maximum 25 mg bid should be added for long-term CHF management if there is no contraindication to β-blockers (do not add β-blockers in acutely ill patients).
- Add digoxin (*Lanoxin*) [T: 0.125, 0.25; S: 0.05 mg/mL]; (*Lanoxicaps*) [T: 0.05, 0.1, 0.2], 0.125–0.375 mg qd (monitor serum levels) if CHF is not controlled on diuretics and ACE inhibitors.
- For patients with NYHA Class III or IV failure and creatinine < 2.5 mg/dL, addition of spironolactone (*Aldactone*) 25 mg qd [T: 25] can reduce mortality; follow serum potassium.
- An angiotensin II receptor blocker is indicated in patients being treated with a diuretic, a β-blocker, and digoxin and who cannot receive an ACE inhibitor secondary to cough or angioedema.
- Some clinicians recommend anticoagulating patients with EF < 25% (see **Table 9**).
- Calcium channel blockers, class I antiarrhythmics, hydralazine, and nitroglycerin are not indicated.
• Diastolic dysfunction:
  - Diuretics should be used judiciously and only if there is volume overload.
  - There is no agreed-upon primary treatment of diastolic dysfunction. β-Blockers, ACE inhibitors, and/or non-dihydropyridine calcium channel blockers may be of benefit.

* Source: Hunt SA, Baker DW, Chin MH, et al. ACC/AHA guidelines for the evaluation and management of chronic heart failure in the adult: executive summary: a report of the American College of Cardiology/American Heart Association Task Force on Practice Guidelines (Committee to Revise the 1995 Guidelines for Evaluation and Management of Heart Failure). *Circulation* 2001;104:2996–3007.

DYSLIPIDEMIA
Treatment Indications
• Older adults should have dyslipidemia treated if they have overt atherosclerotic disease: CHD (angina, previous MI), peripheral arterial disease, abdominal aortic aneurysm, or symptomatic carotid artery disease (TIA or prior stroke). Treatment goal is LDL < 100 mg/dL.
• National Cholesterol Education Program recommends treating diabetes mellitus as CHD risk equivalent. Treatment goal is LDL < 100 mg/dL.
• Dyslipidemia treatment should be considered in older adults without overt atherosclerotic disease or diabetes, but with multiple other CHD risk factors (HTN, smoking, family hx of premature CHD, HDL < 40 mg/dL, male sex). In general, treatment goals are LDL < 130 mg/dL for 2+ risk factors and < 160 mg/dL for 0–1 risk factors. However, more severe individual risk factor profiles may indicate the need for a lower LDL level treatment goal. See http://www.nhlbi.nih.gov.

Management
Nonpharmacologic: A cholesterol-lowering diet should be considered initial therapy for dyslipidemia and should be used as follows:
• The patient should be at low risk for malnutrition.

- The diet should be nutritionally adequate, with sufficient total calories, protein, calcium, iron, and vitamins.
- The diet should be easily understood and affordable (a dietitian can be very helpful).
- Cholesterol-lowering margarines can lower LDL cholesterol by 10% to 15% (*Take Control* 1–2 tablespoons/d; *Benecol* 3 servings of 1.5 teaspoons ea/d).

Pharmacologic: Target drug treatment according to type of dyslipidemia.

Table 15. Drug Regimens for Dyslipidemia			
Condition	**Drug**	**Dosage**	**Formulations**
Elevated LDL, normal TG	HMG-CoA reductase inhibitor*		
	Atorvastatin (*Lipitor*)	10–80 mg qd	[T: 10, 20, 40, 80]
	Fluvastatin (*Lescol*)	20–80 mg qd in PM, max 80 mg	[C: 20, 40; T: ER 80]
	Lovastatin (*Mevacor*)	10–40 mg qd–bid	[T: 10, 20, 40]
	Pravastatin (*Pravachol*)	10–40 mg qd	[T: 10, 20, 40, 80]
	Simvastatin (*Zocor*)	5–80 mg qd in PM	[T: 5, 10, 20, 40, 80]
Elevated TG (> 500 mg/dL)	Gemfibrozil (*Lopid*)	300–600 mg po bid	[T: 600]
Combined elevated LDL, low HDL, elevated TG	Gemfibrozil, HMG-CoA (if TG < 300 mg/dL), conjugated estrogen (in women, see **Table 78**)	as above	as above
Alternative for any of above	Niacin†	100 mg tid to start; increase to 500–1000 mg tid; extended release 150 mg qhs to start, increase to 2000 mg qhs as needed	[T: 25, 50, 100, 250, 500, ER 150, 250, 500, 750, 1000; C: TR 125, 250, 400, 500]
Elevated LDL or combined with inadequate response to one agent	Lovastatin/niacin combination*† (*Advicor*)	20 mg/500 mg qhs to start; increase to 40 mg/ 2000 mg as needed	[T: 20/500, 20/750, 20/1000]

* Baseline CPK and transaminases. Repeat CPK if symptoms of myopathy. Repeat transaminases at 3 mo, then periodically. Watch for myopathy at higher doses or when used with another antidyslipidemic drug. Should be taken in the evening.
† Monitor for flushing, pruritus, nausea, gastritis, ulcer. Dosage increases should be spaced 1 mo apart. ASA 325 mg po 30 min prior to first niacin dose of the day is quite effective in preventing side effects.

HYPERTENSION
Definition, Classification
JNC-VI defines HTN as SBP > 140 or DBP > 90. In elderly persons, many clinicians define HTN as SBP > 160 or DBP > 90. Isolated systolic HTN (SBP > 160 with DBP < 90) should be vigorously treated.

Evaluation and Assessment
• Measure both standing and sitting BP after 5 min of rest.
• Base diagnosis on two or more readings at each of two or more visits. Once diagnosis
  is made, evaluation includes:
  - Assessment of cardiac risk factors: smoking, dyslipidemia, and diabetes mellitus are
    important in older adults.
  - Assessment of end-organ damage: LVH, angina, prior MI, prior coronary
    revascularization, CHF, stroke or TIA, nephropathy, peripheral arterial disease,
    retinopathy.
  - Routine laboratory tests: CBC, UA, electrolytes, creatinine, fasting glucose, total
    cholesterol, HDL cholesterol, and ECG.
  - Think renal artery stenosis if sudden onset of HTN, sudden rise in BP in previously
    well-controlled HTN, or HTN despite treatment with three antihypertensives.

Aggravating Factors
Almost all are related to life style:
• Emotional stress
• Excessive alcohol intake
• Excessive salt intake
• Lack of aerobic exercise
• Low potassium intake
• Low calcium intake
• Nicotine
• Obesity

Management
(JNC-VI recommendations.) Target is <140/90 (130/80 in diabetic persons). Lowering BP
below 120/80 is not recommended.
Nonpharmacologic:
• Adequate calcium and magnesium intake as well as a low-fat diet are recommended
  for optimizing general health.
• Adequate dietary potassium intake; fruits and vegetables are the best sources.
• Aerobic exercise—30–45 min most days of the week—is recommended.
• Moderation of alcohol intake—limit to 1 oz of ethanol/d.
• Moderation of dietary sodium: watch for volume depletion with diuretic use.
• Smoking cessation
• Weight reduction in obese persons: even a 10-lb weight loss can significantly
  lower BP.
Pharmacologic:
Table 16 lists commonly used antihypertensives.
• Use antihypertensives carefully in patients with orthostatic BP drop.
• Base treatment decisions on standing BP.
• In the absence of coexisting conditions, a thiazide diuretic or β-blocker can be used
  as a first-line drug.
• In the presence of coexisting conditions, therapy should be individualized
  (see **Table 17**).
• Antihypertensive combinations are listed in **Table 18**.
• Available dose formulations of oral potassium supplements: [T: (mEq) 6, 7, 8, 10, 20; S:
  (mEq/15 mL) 20, 40; powders (mEq/pk) l5, 20, 25]

Hypertensive Emergencies and Urgencies:
- Elevated BP alone without symptoms or target end organ damage rarely requires emergent BP lowering.
- Conditions requiring emergent BP lowering include hypertensive encephalopathy, intracranial hemorrhage, unstable angina, acute MI, acute LV failure with pulmonary edema, dissecting aortic aneurysm.
- Most common initial treatment for emergent BP lowering is sodium nitroprusside (*Nipride*) 0.25–10 mg/kg/min as IV infusion.
- For nonemergent (ie, urgent) BP lowering, give a standard dose of a recommended antihypertensive orally (see **Table 16**) or an extra dose of the patient's usual oral antihypertensive.

Table 16. Oral Antihypertensive Agents			
Class, Drug	**Geriatric Dose Range, total mg/d (times/d)**	**Formulations**	**Comments (Metabolism, Excretion)**
Diuretics			↓ potassium, Na, magnesium levels; ↑ uric acid, calcium, cholesterol (mild), and glucose (mild) levels
Thiazides			
√ Chlorthalidone (*Hygroton*)	12.5–25 (1)	[T: 15, 25, 50, 100]	↑ side effects at > 25 mg/d (L)
√ HCTZ (*Esidrix, HydroDIURIL, Oretic*)	12.5–25 (1)	[T: 25, 50, 100; S: 50 mg/mL; C: 12.5]	↑ side effects at > 25 mg/d (L)
√ Indapamide (*Lozol*)	0.625–2.5 (1)	[T: 1.25, 2.5]	Less or no hypercholesterolemia (L)
√ Metolazone (*Mykrox*)	0.25–0.5 (1)	[T rapid: 0.5]	Monitor electrolytes carefully (L)
√ Metolazone (*Zaroxolyn*)	2.5–5 (1)	[T: 2.5, 5, 10]	Monitor electrolytes carefully (L)
Loop diuretics			
♥ Bumetanide (*Bumex*)	0.5–4 (1–3)	[T: 0.5, 1, 2]	Short duration of action, no hypercalcemia (K)
♥ Furosemide (*Lasix*)	20–160 (1–2)	[T: 20, 40, 80; S: 10, 40 mg/5 mL]	Short duration of action, no hypercalcemia (K)
♥ Torsemide (*Demadex*)	2.5–50 (1–2)	[T: 5, 10, 20, 100]	Short duration of action, no hypercalcemia (K)
Potassium-sparing drugs			
Amiloride (*Midamor*)	2.5–10 (1)	[T: 5]	(L, K)
♥ Spironolactone (*Aldactone*)	12.5–50 (1–2)	[T: 25, 50, 100]	Gynecomastia; appropriate at 25 mg dose in NYHA Class III or IV CHF (L, K)
Triamterene (*Dyrenium*)	25–100 (1–2)	[T: 50, 100]	(L, K)

Note: Listing of side effects is not exhaustive, and side effects are for the class of drugs except where noted for individual drugs. √ = preferred for treating older persons; ♥ = useful in treating heart failure.

(*continues*)

Table 16. Oral Antihypertensive Agents (cont.)

Class, Drug	Geriatric Dose Range, total mg/d (times/d)	Formulations	Comments (Metabolism, Excretion)
Adrenergic Inhibitors			
α-Blockers			Avoid as primary therapy for HTN unless patient has BPH
Doxazosin (*Cardura*)	1–16 (1)	[T: 1, 2, 4, 8]	(L)
Prazosin (*Minipress*)	1–30 (2–3)	[T: 1, 2, 5]	(L)
Terazosin (*Hytrin*)	1–20 (1)	[T: 1, 2, 5, 10; C: 1, 2, 5, 10]	(L, K)
Peripheral agents			
Guanadrel (*Hylorel*)	5–50 (2)	[T: 10, 25]	Postural hypotension, diarrhea (K)
Guanethidine (*Ismelin*)	5–25 (1)	[T: 10, 25]	Postural hypotension, diarrhea (L, K)
Reserpine (*Serpasil*)	0.05–0.25 (1)	[T: 0.1, 0.25]	Sedation, depression, nasal congestion, activation of peptic ulcer (L, K)
Central α-agonists			Sedation, dry mouth, bradycardia, withdrawal hypertension
Clonidine (*Catapres*, *Catapres-TTS*)	0.1–1.2 (2–3) *or* 1 patch/wk	[T: 0.1, 0.2, 0.3; patch: 0.1, 0.2, 0.3 mg/d]	(L, K)
Guanabenz (*Wytensin*)	4–16 (2)	[T: 4, 8]	(L, K)
Guanfacine (*Tenex*)	0.5–2 (1)	[T: 1, 2]	(K)
Methyldopa (*Aldomet*)	250–2500 (2)	[T: 125, 250, 500; S: 250 mg/5 mL]	(L, K)
β-Blockers			Bronchospasm, bradycardia, acute heart failure, may mask insulin-induced hypoglycemia; lipid solubility is a risk factor for delirium
√ Acebutolol (*Sectral*)	200–800 (1)	[C: 200, 400]	β₁, low lipid solubility, intrinsic sympathomimetic activity (L, K)
√ Atenolol (*Tenormin*)	12.5–100 (1)	[T: 25, 50, 100]	β₁, low lipid solubility (K)
√ Betaxolol (*Kerlone*)	5–20 (1)	[T: 10, 20]	β₁, low lipid solubility, intrinsic sympathomimetic activity (L, K)
√ ♥ Bisoprolol (*Zebeta*)	2.5–10 (1)	[T: 5, 10]	β₁, low lipid solubility (L, K)
√ Carteolol (*Cartrol*)	1.25–10 (1)	[T: 2.5, 5]	β₁, low lipid solubility, intrinsic sympathomimetic activity (K)
√ Metoprolol (*Lopressor*)	25–400 (2)	[T: 25, 50, 100]	β₁, moderate lipid solubility (L)
√ ♥ Long-acting (*Toprol XL*)	50–400 (1)	[T: 25, 50, 100, 200]	(L)
Nadolol (*Corgard*)	20–160 (1)	[T: 20, 40, 80, 120, 160]	β₁, β₂, low lipid solubility (K)
Penbutolol (*Levatol*)	10–20 (1)	[T: 20]	β₁, β₂, high lipid solubility (L, K)

Note: Listing of side effects is not exhaustive, and side effects are for the class of drugs except where noted for individual drugs. √ = preferred for treating older persons; ♥ = useful in treating heart failure.

Class, Drug	Geriatric Dose Range, total mg/d (times/d)	Formulations	Comments (Metabolism, Excretion)
Pindolol (*Visken*)	5–60 (2)	[T: 5, 10]	β_1, β_2, moderate lipid solubility, intrinsic sympathomimetic activity (K)
Propranolol (*Inderal*)	20–360 (2)	[T: 10, 20, 40, 60, 80, 90; S: 4 mg/mL, 8 mg/mL, 80 mg/mL]	β_1, β_2, high lipid solubility (L)
Long-acting (*Inderal LA*)	60–320 (1)	[C: 60, 80, 120, 160]	β_1, β_2, high lipid solubility (L)
Timolol (*Blocadren*)	10–60 (2)	[T: 5, 10, 20]	β_1, β_2, low to moderate lipid solubility (L, K)
Combined α- and β-Blockers			Postural hypotension, bronchospasm
√ ♥ Carvedilol (*Coreg*)	3.125–25 (2)	[T: 3.125, 6.25, 12.5, 25]	β_1, β_2, high lipid solubility (L)
√ Labetalol (*Normodyne, Trandate*)	100–600 (2)	[T: 100, 200, 300]	β_1, β_2, moderate lipid solubility (L, K)
Direct Vasodilators			Headaches, fluid retention, tachycardia
Hydralazine (*Apresoline*)	40–200 (2–4)	[T: 10, 25, 50, 100]	Lupus syndrome (L, K)
Minoxidil (*Loniten*)	2.5–50 (1)	[T: 2.5, 10]	Hirsutism (K)
Calcium Antagonists			
Nondihydropyridines			Conduction defects, worsening of systolic dysfunction, gingival hyperplasia
√ Diltiazem SR (*Cardizem CD, Cardizem SR, Dilacor XR, Tiazac*)	120–360 (1–2) max 480	[C: 1/d: 120, 180, 240, 300, 360, 420; 2/d: 60, 90, 120; T: 30, 60, 90, 120, ER: 120, 180, 240]	Nausea, headache (L)
√ Verapamil SR (*Calan SR, Covera-HS, Isoptin SR, Verelan*)	120–480 (1–2)	[T: SR 120, 180, 240; C: SR 100, 120, 180, 200, 240, 300, 360; T: 40, 80, 120]	Constipation, bradycardia (L)
Dihydropyridines			Ankle edema, flushing, headache, gingival hypertrophy
√ Amlodipine (*Norvasc*)	2.5–10 (1)	[T: 2.5, 5, 10]	(L)
√ Felodipine (*Plendil*)	2.5–20 (1)	[T: 2.5, 5, 10]	(L)
√ Isradipine (*DynaCirc*)	5–20 (2)	[T: 2.5, 5]	(L)
√ Sustained release (*DynaCirc CR*)	5–20 (1)	[T: 5, 10]	

Note: Listing of side effects is not exhaustive, and side effects are for the class of drugs except where noted for individual drugs. √ = preferred for treating older persons; ♥ = useful in treating heart failure.

(*continues*)

Table 16. Oral Antihypertensive Agents (cont.)			
Class, Drug	Geriatric Dose Range, total mg/d (times/d)	Formulations	Comments (Metabolism, Excretion)
√ Nicardipine (*Cardene*)	60–120 (3)	[C: 20, 30]	(L)
√ Sustained release (*Cardene SR*)	60–120 (2)	[T: 30, 45, 60]	(L)
√ Nifedipine SR (*Adalat CC, Procardia XL*)	30–120 (1)	[T: 30, 60, 90]	(L)
√ Nisoldipine (*Sular*)	20–60 (1)	[T: ER 10, 20, 30, 40]	(L)
ACE Inhibitors			Cough (common), angioedema (rare), hyperkalemia, rash, loss of taste, leukopenia
√ ♥ Benazepril (*Lotensin*)	2.5–40 (1–2)	[T: 5, 10, 20, 40]	(L, K)
√ ♥ Captopril (*Capoten*)	12.5–150 (2–3)	[T: 12.5, 25, 50, 100]	(L, K)
√ ♥ Enalapril (*Vasotec*)	2.5–40 (1–2)	[T: 2.5, 5, 10, 20]	(L, K)
√ ♥ Fosinopril (*Monopril*)	5–40 (1–2)	[T: 10, 20, 40]	(L, K)
√ ♥ Lisinopril (*Prinivil, Zestril*)	2.5–40 (1)	[T: 2.5, 5, 10, 20, 30, 40]	(K)
√ ♥ Moexipril (*Univasc*)	3.75–15 (2)	[T: 7.5, 15]	(L, K)
√ ♥ Perindopril (*Aceon*)	4–8 (1–2)	[T: 2, 4, 8]	(L, K)
√ ♥ Quinapril (*Accupril*)	5–80 (1–2)	[T: 5, 10, 20, 40]	(L, K)
√ ♥ Ramipril (*Altace*)	1.25–20 (1–2)	[T: 1.25, 2.5, 5, 10]	(L, K)
√ ♥ Trandolapril (*Mavik*)	1–4 (1)	[T: 1, 2, 4]	(L, K)
Angiotensin II Receptor Blockers (ARBs)			Angioedema (very rare), hyperkalemia
√ ♥ Candesartan (*Atacand*)	4–32 (1)	[T: 4, 8, 16, 32]	(K)
√ ♥ Eprosartan (*Teveten*)	400–800 (1–2)	[T: 400, 600]	(biliary, K)
√ ♥ Irbesartan (*Avapro*)	75–300 (1)	[T: 75, 150, 300]	(L)
√ ♥ Losartan (*Cozaar*)	12.5–100 (1–2)	[T: 25, 50, 100]	(L, K)
√ ♥ Olmesartan (*Benicar*)	20–40 (1)	[T: 5, 20, 40]	(F, K)
√ ♥ Telmisartan (*Micardis*)	20–80 (1)	[T: 20, 40, 80]	(L)
√ ♥ Valsartan (*Diovan*)	40–320 (1)	[T: 80, 160, 320; C: 80, 160]	(L, K)

Note: Listing of side effects is not exhaustive, and side effects are for the class of drugs except where noted for individual drugs. √ = preferred for treating older persons; ♥ = useful in treating heart failure.
Source: Data in part from JNC-VI: the sixth report of the Joint National Committee on Prevention, Detection, Evaluation, and Treatment of High Blood Pressure. *Arch Intern Med.* 1997;157:2413-2446.

Table 17. Choosing Antihypertensive Therapy on the Basis of Coexisting Conditions		
Condition	Appropriate For Use	Avoid or Contraindicated
Angina	β, D, non-D	
Atrial tachycardia and fibrillation	β, non-D	
Bronchospasm		β, αβ
CHF	ACEI, ARB, β, αβ, L	D, non-D*

Table 17. Choosing Antihypertensive Therapy on the Basis of Coexisting Conditions (cont.)

Condition	Appropriate For Use	Avoid or Contraindicated
Depression		β
Diabetes mellitus	ACEI, β, T†	T†
Dyslipidemia		β, T†
Essential tremor	β	
Hyperthyroidism	β	
MI	β, ACEI	non-D
Osteoporosis	T	
Prostatism (BPH)	α	
Renal insufficiency	ACEI§	
Urge UI	D, non-D	L, T

Note: α = α-blocker; β = β-blocker; αβ = combined α- and β-blocker; ACEI = ACE inhibitor; ARB = angiotensin receptor blocker; D = dihydropyridine calcium antagonist; non-D = nondihydropyridine calcium antagonist; L = loop diuretic; T = thiazide diuretic.

* May be beneficial in CHF caused by diastolic dysfunction.

† Low-dose diuretics are probably beneficial in type 2 diabetes; high-dose diuretics are relatively contraindicated in types 1 and 2.

† Low-dose diuretics have a minimal effect on lipids.

§ Use with great caution in renovascular disease.

Table 18. Antihypertensive Combinations

Drug	Trade Name
β-Adrenergic Blockers and Diuretics	
Atenolol, 50 or 100 mg *with* chlorthalidone, 25 mg	*Tenoretic*
Bisoprolol fumarate, 2.5, 5, or 10 mg *with* HCTZ, 6.25 mg	*Ziac*
Metoprolol tartrate, 50 or 100 mg *with* HCTZ, 25 or 50 mg	*Lopressor HCT*
Nadolol, 40 or 80 mg *with* bendroflumethiazide, 5 mg	*Corzide*
Propranolol hydrochloride, 40 or 80 mg *with* HCTZ, 25 mg	*Inderide*
Propranolol hydrochloride (extended release), 80, 120, or 160 mg *with* HCTZ, 50	*Inderide LA*
Timolol maleate, 10 mg *with* HCTZ, 25 mg	*Timolide*
ACE Inhibitors and Diuretics	
Benazepril hydrochloride, 5, 10, or 20 mg *with* HCTZ, 6.25, 12.5, or 25 mg	*Lotensin HTC*
Captopril, 25 or 50 mg *with* HCTZ, 15 or 25 mg	*Capozide*
Enalapril maleate, 5 or 10 mg *with* HCTZ, 12.5 or 25 mg	*Vaseretic*
Fosinopril, 10 or 20 mg *with* HCTZ, 12.5 mg	*Monopril HCT*
Lisinopril, 10 or 20 mg *with* HCTZ, 12.5 or 25 mg	*Prinzide, Zestoretic*
Moexipril, 7.5 or 15 mg *with* HCTZ, 12.5; also 15 mg *with* HCTZ, 25 mg	*Uniretic*
Angiotensin II Receptor Blockers and Diuretics	
Candesartan, 16, 32 mg *with* HCTZ, 12.5 mg	*Atacand-HCT*
Losartan potassium, 50 or 100 mg *with* HCTZ, 12.5 or 25 mg	*Hyzaar*
Irbesartan, 150 or 300 mg *with* HCTZ, 12.5 mg	*Avalide*
Telmisartan, 40, 80 mg *with* HCTZ, 12.5 mg	*Micardis-HCT*
Valsartan, 80 mg *with* HCTZ, 12.5 mg; also 160 mg *with* HCTZ, 25 mg	*Diovan-HCT*
Calcium Antagonists and ACE Inhibitors	
Amlodipine besylate, 2.5, 5, or 10 mg *with* benazepril hydrochloride, 10 or 20 mg	*Lotrel*

(*continues*)

Table 18. Antihypertensive Combinations (cont.)	
Drug	**Trade Name**
Diltiazem hydrochloride, 180 mg *with* enalapril maleate, 5 mg	*Teczem*
Felodipine, 5 mg *with* enalapril maleate, 5 mg	*Lexxel*
Verapamil hydrochloride (extended release), 180 or 240 mg *with* trandolapril, 1, 2, or 4 mg	*Tarka*
Other Combinations	
Amiloride hydrochloride, 5 mg *with* HCTZ, 50 mg	*Moduretic*
Clonidine hydrochloride, 0.1, 0.2, or 0.3 mg *with* chlorthalidone, 15 mg	*Combipres*
Hydralazine hydrochloride, 25, 50, or 100 mg *with* HCTZ, 25 or 50 mg	*Apresazide*
Guanethidine monosulfate, 10 mg *with* HCTZ, 25 mg	*Esimil*
Methyldopa, 250 mg *with* chlorothiazide, 150 or 250 mg	*Aldoclor*
Methyldopa, 250 or 500 mg *with* HCTZ, 15, 25, 30, or 50 mg	*Aldoril*
Prazosin hydrochloride, 1, 2, or 5 mg *with* polythiazide, 0.5 mg	*Minizide*
Reserpine, 0.125 or 0.25 mg *with* chlorothiazide, 250 or 500 mg	*Diupres*
Reserpine, 0.125 or 0.25 mg *with* chlorthalidone, 25 or 50 mg	*Demi-Regroton*
Reserpine, 0.10 mg *with* hydralazine hydrochloride, 25 mg *with* HCTZ, 15 mg	*Ser-Ap-Es*
Reserpine, 0.125 mg *with* HCTZ, 25 or 50 mg	*Hydropres*
Spironolactone, 25 or 50 mg *with* HCTZ, 25 or 50 mg	*Aldactazide*
Triamterene, 37.5, 50, or 75 mg *with* HCTZ, 25 or 50 mg	*Dyazide, Maxzide*

Source: JNC-VI: the sixth report of the Joint National Committee on Prevention, Detection, Evaluation, and Treatment of High Blood Pressure. *Arch Intern Med.* 1997;157:2427.

ATRIAL FIBRILLATION
Evaluation and Assessment
Causes:
- Cardiac disease: Cardiac surgery, cardiomyopathy, CHF, hypertensive heart disease, ischemic disease, pericarditis, valvular disease
- Noncardiac disease: Alcoholism, chronic pulmonary disease, infections, pulmonary emboli, thyrotoxicosis
- Standard testing: ECG, CXR, CBC, electrolytes, creatinine, BUN, TSH, echocardiogram

Management
- Correct precipitating cause(s).
- Acute-onset:
  - D/C cardioversion if compromised cardiac output or angina
  - If hemodynamically stable with rapid ventricular response (> 100 beats/min), lower ventricular rate medically. Options include:
    β-blockers (eg, atenolol [*Tenormin*] 5 mg IV over 5 min, may repeat in 10 min [0.5 mg/mL], followed by 25–100 mg po qd [T: 25, 50, 100]);
    calcium channel blockers (eg, diltiazem [*Cardizem injectable*] 20 mg IV bolus, giving 25 mg IV 15 min later if necessary, with a maintenance infusion of 5–15 mg/h, followed by 120–360 mg po qd of long-acting preparation [*Cardizem CD, Dilacor XR*; T: 120, 180, 240, 300, 360].
    Although it works more slowly for rate control, digoxin [*Lanoxin*] is another option: 0.25 mg IV q 6 h up to 0.75 mg [0.05 mg/mL], followed by 0.125–0.25 mg po qd [T: 0.125, 0.25].

- If electric cardioversion or lowering of ventricular rate has not converted patient to sinus rhythm, begin anticoagulation with IV unfractionated heparin (see **Table 11**) followed by oral warfarin (see p 17); seek cardiology consultation for possible electric or pharmacologic cardioversion.
- Chronic AF:
  - Anticoagulate (see **Table 9**) if there are no contraindications.
  - If anticoagulation is contraindicated, begin ASA 325 mg po qd.
  - If electric cardioversion has not been tried in the past, seek cardiology consultation for possible cardioversion.
  - Rate control (goal < 80/min averaged over 1 h) can be achieved with oral β-blockers, calcium channel blockers, or digoxin (see above for examples and dosages).

AORTIC STENOSIS (AS)
Evaluation and Assessment
- Presence of symptoms—angina, syncope, CHF (frequently diastolic dysfunction)—indicates severe disease and a life expectancy without surgery of < 2 yr.
- Echocardiography is essential in the work-up to measure aortic jet velocity (AJV) and aortic valve area (AVA).
  - Moderate AS is indicated by an AJV of 3.0–4.0 meters/sec and by an AVA of 1.0–1.5 cm^2.
  - Severe AS is indicated by an AJV > 4.0 meters/sec and by an AVA < 1.0 cm^2.
- For asymptomatic cases, echocardiography should be repeated annually for moderate AS and every 6–12 mo for severe AS.
- ECG and CXR should be obtained initially to look for conduction defects, LVH, and pulmonary congestion.

Treatment
- Aortic valve replacement (AVR) surgery
  - Alleviates symptoms and improves ventricular functioning.
  - In most cases, AVR should be performed promptly *after* symptoms have appeared.
  - Risks and benefits of AVR should be considered on individual basis (see pp 126–127).
- There is no effective medical treatment. Vasodilators should be avoided if possible.

PERIPHERAL ARTERIAL DISEASE

Table 19. Classes of Peripheral Arterial Disease			
Class	**ABI**	**Symptoms**	**Treatment**
Normal	> 0.9	None	RFM
Mild	0.8–0.9	No limitation in walking distance	RFM, AT
Moderate to severe	0.4–0.8	Walking limited by claudication	RFM, AT, CRx
Severe to critical	< 0.4	Rest pain; ischemia on exam	RFM, AT, CRx, LS

Note: ABI = ankle-brachial BP index; AT = antiplatelet therapy; CRx = claudication therapy; LS = limb salvage; RFM = risk factor modification.

Treatment
Risk Factor Modification:
- Low-fat diet
- Exercise: walking program
- Smoking cessation
- Lipid-lowering therapy
- BP control
- Glycemic control in diabetic patients

Antiplatelet Therapy:
- ASA 325 mg qd
- Clopidogrel (*Plavix*) 75 mg qd [T: 75] if ASA failure or intolerant to ASA

Claudication Treatment:
- Walking program
- Drug therapy: cilostazol (*Pletal*) 100 mg bid (contraindicated in patients with CHF) 1 h before or 2 h after meals [T: 50, 100]; pentoxifylline (*Trental*) 400 mg tid [T: 400]; conventional analgesics

Limb Salvage:
- Percutaneous angioplasty
- Bypass surgery

DELIRIUM

DIAGNOSIS
Diagnostic Criteria—Adapted from *DSM-IV*
- Disturbed consciousness (ie, decreased attention, environmental awareness)
- Cognitive change (eg, memory deficit, disorientation, language disturbance), or perceptual disturbance (eg, visual illusions, hallucinations)
- Rapid onset (hours to days) and fluctuating daily course
- Evidence of a causal physical condition

Risk Factors
- Dementia greatly increases risk for delirium.
- Advanced age, comorbid physical problems (especially sleep deprivation, immobility, dehydration, sensory impairment.)

Evaluation
- Assume reversibility unless proven otherwise.
- Thoroughly review prescription and OTC medications.
- Exclude infection and other medical causes.
- Laboratory studies may include CBC, electrolytes, LFTs, renal function tests, serum calcium and glucose, UA, oxygen saturation, CXR, and ECG
- Confusion Assessment Method (CAM): BOTH acute onset and fluctuating course AND inattention AND EITHER disorganized thinking OR altered level of consciousness (Inouye S, *Ann Intern Med*. 1990;113:941–948).

CAUSES (* = most common)
Drugs
- Anticholinergics* (eg, diphenhydramine), TCAs, (eg, amitriptyline, imipramine), antipsychotics (eg, chlorpromazine, thioridazine)
- Anti-inflammatory agents, including prednisone
- Benzodiazepines or alcohol—acute toxicity or withdrawal
- Cardiovascular (eg, digitalis, antihypertensives)
- Diuretics
- Lithium
- GI (eg, cimetidine, ranitidine)
- Opioid analgesics (especially meperidine)

Infections
Respiratory*, skin*, urinary tract*, and others

Metabolic Disorders
Acute blood loss, dehydration*, electrolyte imbalance*, end-organ failure (hepatic, renal), hyperglycemia, hypoglycemia*, hypoxia*

Cardiovascular
Arrhythmia, CHF*, MI*, shock

Neurologic
CNS infections, head trauma, seizures, stroke, subdural hematoma, TIAs, tumors

Miscellaneous
Fecal impaction, postoperative state*, sleep deprivation, urinary retention

MANAGEMENT
Nonpharmacologic
- Identify and remove or treat underlying cause(s)
- Provide general supportive measures:
  - Environmental modifications
       communication to reorient to new surroundings
       objects that provide orientation (eg, calendar, clock)
       quiet, well-lit surroundings (eg, night lights)
       familiar faces (eg, family members) at bedside for reassurance
       sitters
  - Stimulating activities during daytime
       cognitive activities (eg, current events discussion, word games)
       ambulation, active range-of-motion exercises
  - Correction of sensory deficits
       eyeglasses
       adequate lighting
       magnifying lenses
       cerumen removal
       hearing aids
       portable amplification device
  - Measures to promote normal sleep
       warm milk at bedtime
       relaxation tapes
       back massage
       nighttime noise reduction
  - Prevention of dehydration
       oral or parenteral supplementation if BUN/creatinine ratio > 18
  - Physical restraints (only as last resort to maintain patient safety, eg, preventing
    patient from pulling out tubes or catheters)

Pharmacologic
- For acute agitation or aggression accompanying delirium, use a high-potency
  antipsychotic such as haloperidol (*Haldol*) 0.5–2 mg po [T: 0.5, 1, 2, 5, 10, 20;
  S: 2 mg/mL] or IV or IM (twice as potent as po). May also be given as slow IV push;
  titrate upward as needed. Reevaluate every 30 min. Observe for development of EPS.
  Avoid low-potency antipsychotics such as chlorpromazine (*Thorazine*) or thioridazine
  (*Mellaril*) because of their anticholinergic and arrythmogenic properties (torsade de
  pointes). If patient is able to take drugs po, consider low dose of atypical antipsychotic
  (see **Table 64**).
- If delirium is secondary to alcohol or benzodiazepine withdrawal, use a
  benzodiazepine such as lorazepam (*Ativan*) in doses of 0.5–2 mg every 4–6 h. Since
  these agents themselves may cause delirium, gradual withdrawal and discontinuation
  are desirable. If delirium is secondary to alcohol, also use thiamine 100 mg qd (po, IM,
  or IV).

DEMENTIA

DEMENTIA SYNDROME
Definition
Acquired decline in memory and in at least one other cognitive function (eg, language, visual-spatial, executive) sufficient to affect daily life in an alert person.

Estimated Frequencies of Dementia Causes
- AD: 60% to 70%
- Other progressive disorders: 15% to 30% (eg, vascular, Lewy body)
- Completely reversible dementia (eg, drug toxicity, metabolic changes, thyroid disease, subdural hematoma, normal-pressure hydrocephalus): 2% to 5%

DIAGNOSIS OF AD
- Dementia syndrome
- Gradual onset and continuing decline
- Not due to another physical, neurologic, or psychiatric condition or to medications
- Deficits not occurring exclusively during delirium

PROGRESSION OF AD

Mild Cognitive Impairment   (preclinical)   MMSE: 26–30
- Delayed paragraph recall
- Cognition otherwise intact
- No functional impairment
- Mild construction, language, or executive dysfunction

Early, Mild Impairment   (yr 1–3 from onset of symptoms)   MMSE: 22–28
- Disorientation for date
- Naming difficulties (anomia)
- Recent recall problems
- Mild difficulty copying figures
- Decreased insight
- Social withdrawal
- Irritability, mood change
- Problems managing finances

Middle, Moderate Impairment   (yr 2–8)   MMSE: 10–21
- Disoriented to date, place
- Comprehension difficulties (aphasia)
- Impaired new learning
- Getting lost in familiar areas
- Impaired calculating skills
- Delusions, agitation, aggression
- Not cooking, shopping, banking
- Restless, anxious, depressed
- Problems with dressing, grooming

Late, Severe Impairment   (yr 6–12)   MMSE: 0–9
- Nearly unintelligible verbal output
- Remote memory gone
- Unable to copy or write
- No longer grooming or dressing
- Incontinent
- Motor or verbal agitation

NONCOGNITIVE SYMPTOMS

Psychotic Symptoms (eg, Delusions, Hallucinations)
- Occur in about one third of AD patients
- Delusions may be paranoid (eg, people stealing things, spouse unfaithful)
- Hallucinations more commonly visual

Depressive Symptoms
- Occur in up to 40% of AD patients; may herald onset of AD
- May cause acceleration of decline if untreated
- Need to suspect if patient stops eating or withdraws

Agitation or Aggression
- Occurs in up to 80% of patients with AD
- A leading cause of nursing-home admission
- Consider superimposed delirium or pain as a trigger

RISK AND PROTECTIVE FACTORS FOR AD

Definite Risks	Possible Risks	Possible Protections
Age	Other genes	Estrogen
Family history	Head trauma	NSAIDs
Down syndrome	Lower educational level	Antioxidants
APOE-E4	Depression	

Clinical Features Distinguishing AD and Other Types of Dementia
- AD: Memory, language, visual-spatial disturbances, indifference, delusions, agitation
- Frontotemporal dementia: Personality change, executive dysfunction, hyperorality, relative preservation of visual-spatial skills
- Lewy body dementia: visual hallucinations, delusions, extrapyramidal symptoms, fluctuating mental status, sensitivity to antipsychotic medications

EVALUATION
Although completely reversible (eg, drug toxicity) dementia is rare, identifying and treating secondary physical conditions may improve function.
- History: Obtain from family or other informant
- Physical and neurologic examination
- Assess functional status
- Evaluate mental status for attention, immediate and delayed recall, remote memory, executive function, and depression. Screening tests may include Mini-Cog (p 170), number of animals named in 1 min, MMSE, GDS (p 172)

Laboratory Testing
CBC, TSH, B_{12}, serum calcium, liver and renal function tests, electrolytes, serologic test for syphilis (selectively); at this time genetic testing and commercial "Alzheimer blood tests" are not recommended for clinical use.

Neuroimaging
The likelihood of detecting structural lesions is increased with:
- Onset age < 60
- Focal (unexplained) neurologic signs or symptoms

• Abrupt onset or rapid decline (weeks to months)
• Predisposing conditions (eg, metastatic cancer or anticoagulants)

Neuroimaging may detect the 5% of patients with clinically significant structural lesions that would otherwise be missed.

TREATMENT
Primary goals of treatment are to improve quality of life and maximize functional performance by enhancing cognition, mood, and behavior.

General Treatment Principles
• Identify and treat comorbid physical illnesses (eg, HTN, diabetes mellitus)
• Set realistic goals
• Limit prn psychotropic medication use
• Specify and quantify target behaviors
• Maximize and maintain functioning

Nonpharmacologic Approaches
To improve function:
• Behavior modification, scheduled toileting, and prompted toileting (see p 161) for UI
• Graded assistance (as little help as possible to perform ADLs), practice, and positive reinforcement to increase independence

For problem behaviors:
• Music during meals, bathing
• Walking or light exercise
• Simulate family presence with video or audio tapes
• Pet therapy
• Speak at patient's comprehension level
• Bright light, white noise

Pharmacologic Treatment of Cognitive Dysfunction in AD
• Patients with a diagnosis of mild or moderate AD should receive a cholinesterase inhibitor that will increase level of acetylcholine in brain (**Table 20**) (demonstrated benefit for cognition, mood, behavioral symptoms, and daily function). Controlled data show benefits of cholinergic drugs for 1 yr and open trials demonstrate benefit for 3 yr. Only 25% of patients taking cholinesterase inhibitors show clinical improvement but 80% have less rapid decline. Initial studies show benefits of these drugs for patients with Lewy body dementia and dementia with vascular risk factors. Prolonged cholinergic therapy may delay nursing-home placement. To evaluate response or stabilize:
    - Elicit caregiver observations of patient's behavior (alertness, initiative) and follow functional status (ADLs and IADLs).
    - Follow cognitive status (eg, improved or stabilized) by caregiver's report or serial ratings of cognition (eg, Mini-Cog, see p 170; MMSE).
• Consider the antioxidant vitamin E at 1000 IU bid (shown to delay functional decline thought to occur from oxidative stress).
• *Ginkgo biloba* is not generally recommended because clinical trial results are not yet definitive, and preparations vary since such nutriceuticals are not FDA regulated.

Table 20. Cholinesterase Inhibitors*		
Drug	**Formulations**	**Dosing (Metabolism)**
Donepezil (*Aricept*)	[T: 5, 10]	Start at 5 mg qd, increase to 10 mg qd after 1 mo (CYP2D6, 3A4) (L)
Galantamine (*Reminyl*)	[T: 4, 8, 12; S: 4 mg/mL]	Start at 4 mg bid, increase to 8 mg bid after 4 wk; recommended dose 16–24 mg/d (CYP2D6, 3A4) (L)
Rivastigmine (*Exelon*)	[T: 1.5, 3, 4.5, 6]	Start at 1.5 mg bid and gradually titrate up to 6 mg bid as tolerated; retitrate if drug is stopped (K)

* Side effects increase with higher dosing. Continue if improvement or stabilization occurs; stopping drugs can lead to rapid decline. Possible side effects include nausea, vomiting, diarrhea, dyspepsia, anorexia, weight loss, leg cramps, bradycardia, and agitation.

Treatment of Agitation

Table 21. Agitation Treatment Guidelines			
Symptom	**Drug**	**Dosage**	**Formulations**
Agitation in context of nonacute psychosis	Risperidone (*Risperdal*)	0.25–1.5 mg/d	[T: 0.25, 0.5, 1, 2, 3, 4; S: 1 mg/mL]
	Olanzapine (*Zyprexa*) (*Zydis*)	2.5–10 mg/d	[T: 2.5, 5, 7.5, 10, 15, 20] [T: orally disintegrating 5, 10, 15, 20]
	Quetiapine (*Seroquel*)	25–400 mg/d	[T: 25, 100, 200, 300]
	Thiothixene (*Navane*)	2–4 mg/d*	[C: 1, 2, 5, 10, 20]
Acute psychosis agitation if IM or IV is needed	Haloperidol (*Haldol*)	0.5–2 mg/d*	[T: 0.5, 1, 2, 5, 10, 20; S: 2 mg/mL; Inj]
Agitation in context of depression	SSRI, eg, citalopram (*Celexa*)	10–30 mg/d	[T: 20, 40; S: 2mg/mL]
Anxiety, mild to moderate irritability	Trazodone (*Desyrel*)	50–100 mg/d†	[T: 50, 100, 150, 300]
	Buspirone (*BuSpar*)	30–60 mg/d‡	[T: 5, 7.5, 10, 15, 30]
As a possible second-line treatment for significant agitation or aggression	Divalproex sodium (*Depakote*)	500–1500 mg/d§	[T: 125, 250, 500; S: syr 250 mg/mL; sprinkle capsule: 125]
	Carbamazepine (*Tegretol*)	300–600 mg/d§§	[T: 200; ChT: 100; S: sus 100/5 mL]
Sexual aggression, impulse-control symptoms in men	Estrogen (*Premarin*) or medroxyprogesterone (*Depo-Provera*)	0.625–1.25 mg/d 100 mg IM/wk	[T: 0.3, 0.625, 0.9, 1.25, 2.5] [Inj]

* May need to give higher doses in emergency situations; should be used for only short periods of time.
† Small divided daytime dosage and larger bedtime dosage; watch for sedation and orthostasis.
‡ Can be given bid; 2–4 wk for adequate trial.
§ Can monitor serum levels; usually well tolerated; check CBC, platelets for agranulocytosis, thrombocytopenia risk in older patients.
§§ Monitor serum levels; periodic CBCs, platelet counts secondary to agranulocytosis risk. Beware of drug-drug interactions.

CAREGIVER ISSUES
- Over 50% develop depression.
- Physical illness, isolation, anxiety, and burnout are common.
- Intensive education and support of caregivers may delay institutionalization.
- Adult day care for patients and respite services may help.
- Alzheimer's Association offers support, education; chapters are located in major cities throughout US. (See p 190 for telephone, Web site.)
- Family Caregiver Alliance offers support, education, information for caregivers. (See p 190 for telephone, Web site.)

REPORT OF THE QUALITY STANDARDS SUBCOMMITTEE OF THE AAN
Doody RS, Stevens JC, Beck C, et al. Practice parameter: management of dementia (an evidence-based review): report of the Quality Standards Subcommittee of the American Academy of Neurology. *Neurology* 2001; 56(9):1154–1166.

EVALUATION AND ASSESSMENT

Recognizing and diagnosing late-life depression can be difficult. Older patients may complain of lack of energy or other somatic symptoms, attribute symptoms to old age or other physical conditions, or fail to mention them to a health care professional.

Medical Evaluation

TSH, B_{12}, calcium, LFTs, renal function tests, electrolytes, UA, CBC

DSM-IV Criteria for Major Depressive Episode (Abbreviated)

Five or more of the following symptoms have been present during the same 2-wk period and represent a change from previous functioning; at least one of the symptoms is either (1) depressed mood or (2) loss of interest or pleasure.

- Depressed mood
- Loss of interest or pleasure in activities
- Significant weight loss or gain (not intentional), or decrease or increase in appetite
- Insomnia or hypersomnia
- Psychomotor agitation or retardation
- Fatigue or loss of energy
- Feelings of worthlessness or excessive or inappropriate guilt
- Diminished ability to think or concentrate, or indecisiveness
- Recurrent thoughts of death, suicidal ideation, attempt, or plan

The *DSM-IV* criteria are not specific for older adults; cognitive symptoms may be more prominent. The GDS and other instruments are useful for screening and monitoring (see p 172).

MANAGEMENT

Treatment should be individualized on the basis of hx, past response, and severity of illness as well as concurrent illnesses. Treatments may be combined.

Nonpharmacologic

For mild to moderate depression or in combination with pharmacotherapy: cognitive-behavioral therapy, interpersonal therapy, problem-solving therapy.

Pharmacologic

For mild, moderate, or severe depression: the duration of therapy should be at least 6–12 mo following remission for patients experiencing their first depressive episode. Most older patients with a hx of major depression require lifelong antidepressant therapy.

Choosing an Antidepressant (see Table 22 and list at top of p 49)

Consider an SSRI: As first-line choice for most older patients, especially:

- Patients with heart conduction defects or ischemic heart disease
- Patients with prostatic hyperplasia
- Patients with uncontrolled glaucoma

Consider Venlafaxine, Mirtazapine, or Bupropion: As second-line choice
Consider Nortriptyline or Desipramine:
• As a third-line treatment for severe melancholic depression
• For patients with urge incontinence, but use tolterodine (*Detrol*) and an SSRI if avoidance of central anticholinergic effects of a TCA is important (see **Table 75**)

Table 22. Antidepressants Used for Older Adults				
Class, Drug	Initial Dosage	Usual Dosage	Formulations	Comments (Metabolism, Excretion)
Selective Serotonin-Reuptake Inhibitors				Class side effects (EPS, hyponatremia) (L, K [10%])
Citalopram (*Celexa*)	10–20 mg qam	20–30 mg/d	[T: 20, 40, 60; S: 5 mg/ 10 mL]	
Escitalopram (*Lexapro*)	10 mg/d	10 mg/d	[T: 5, 10, 20]	Currently limited geriatric experience
Fluoxetine (*Prozac*)	5 mg qam	5–60 mg/d	[T: 10; C: 10, 20, 40; S: 20 mg/5 mL; C: SR 90 (weekly dose)]	Long half-lives of parent and active metabolite may allow for less frequent dosing; CYP2D6, -2C9, -3A4 inhibitor (L)
Fluvoxamine (*Luvox*)	25 mg qhs	100–300 mg/d	[T: 25, 50, 100]	Not approved as an antidepressant in US; CYP1A2, -3A4 inhibitor (L)
Paroxetine (*Paxil*)	5 mg	10–40 mg/d	[T: 10, 20, 30, 40]	Helpful if anxiety symptoms are prominent; CYP2D6 inhibitor (L)
(*Paxil CR*)	12.5 mg/d	—	[T: ER 12.5, 25, 37.5; S: 10 mg/ 5 mL]	Increase by 12.5 mg/d no faster than 1/wk
Sertraline (*Zoloft*)	25 mg qam	50–200 mg/d	[T: 25, 50, 100; S: 20 mg/mL]	(L)
Additional Medications				
Bupropion (*Wellbutrin, Zyban*)	37.5–50 mg bid 100 mg (SR) qd or bid	75–150 mg bid 100–150 mg (SR) bid	[T: 75, 100, SR 100, 150]	Consider for SSRI, TCA nonresponders; safe in CHF; may be stimulating; can lower seizure threshold (L)
Methylphenidate (*Ritalin*)	2.5–5 mg at 7 AM and noon	5–10 mg at 7 AM and noon	[T: 5, 10, 20]	Short-term treatment of depression or apathy in physically ill elderly; used as an adjunct (L)

(*continues*)

Table 22. Antidepressants Used for Older Adults (cont.)				
Class, Drug	Initial Dosage	Usual Dosage	Formulations	Comments (Metabolism, Excretion)
Mirtazapine (*Remeron*)	15 mg qhs	15–45 mg/d	[T: 15, 30, 45]	May increase appetite; sedating; oral disintegrating tablet (SolTab) available (L)
Nefazodone (*Serzone*)	50 mg bid	200–400 mg/d	[T: 50, 100, 150, 200, 250]	May help insomnia; sedating in some patients; CYP3A4 inhibition; hepatoxicity, obtain baseline LFT (L)
Trazodone (*Desyrel*)	25 mg qhs	75–600 mg/d	[T: 50, 100, 150, 300]	Sedation may limit dose; may be used as a hypnotic; ventricular irritability; priapism in men (L)
Venlafaxine (*Effexor*)	25–50 mg bid	75–225 mg/d	[T: 25, 37.5, 50, 75, 100]	Low anticholinergic activity; minimal sedation and hypotension; may increase BP; may be useful when somatic pain present; EPS, hyponatremia (L)
(*Effexor XR*)	75 mg qam	75–225 mg/d	[C: 37.5, 75, 150]	Same as above
Tricyclic Antidepressants				
Desipramine (*Norpramin*)	10–25 mg qhs	50–150 mg/d	[T: 10, 25, 50, 75, 100, 150]	Therapeutic serum level>115 ng/mL (L)
Nortriptyline (*Aventyl, Pamelor*)	10–25 mg qhs	75–150 mg/d	[C: 10, 25, 50, 75; S: 10 mg/ 5 mL]	Therapeutic window (50–150 ng/mL) (L)
Monoamine Oxidase Inhibitors				Hypotension; drug, food interactions (K, L)
Isocarboxazid (*Marplan*)	10 mg bid–tid	10 mg tid	[T: 10]	
Phenelzine (*Nardil*)	15 mg qd	15–60 mg/d	[T: 15]	
Tranylcypromine (*Parnate*)	10 mg bid	20–40 mg/d	[T: 10]	

Antidepressants to Avoid in Older Adults
- Amitriptyline (eg, *Elavil*): anticholinergic, sedating, hypotensive
- Amoxapine (*Asendin*): anticholinergic, sedating, hypotensive; also associated with EPS, tardive dyskinesia, and neuroleptic malignant syndrome
- Doxepin (eg, *Sinequan*): anticholinergic, sedating, hypotensive
- Imipramine (*Tofranil*): anticholinergic, sedating, hypotensive
- Maprotiline(*Ludiomil*): seizures and rashes
- Protriptyline (*Vivactil*): very anticholinergic; can be stimulating
- St. John's wort: decreases effects of digoxin and CYP3A4 substrates; efficacy questioned
- Trimipramine (*Surmontil*): anticholinergic, sedating, hypotensive

Electroconvulsive Therapy
Generally safe and very effective.
Indications: Severe depression when a rapid onset of response is necessary; when depression is resistant to drug therapy; for patients who are unable to tolerate antidepressants, have previous response to ECT, have psychotic depression, severe catatonia, or depression with Parkinson's disease.
Complications: Temporary confusion, arrhythmias, aspiration, falls.
Contraindications:
- Increased intracranial pressure
- Intracranial tumor
- MI within 3 mo (relative)
- Stroke within 1 mo (relative)

Before ECT evaluation: CXR, ECG, serum electrolytes, and cardiac examination. Additional tests (eg, stress test, neuroimaging, EEG) are used selectively.

DERMATOLOGIC CONDITIONS

COMMON DERMATOLOGIC CONDITIONS

Table 23. Dermatologic Conditions Common in Elderly Persons

Condition	Areas Affected	Description
Candidiasis	Body folds	Erythema, pustules, or cheesy, whitish matter, satellite lesions
Treatment: See intertrigo, next; antifungal powders (see list in next section)		
Intertrigo	Any place 2 skin surfaces rest against one another (eg, under the breasts)	Moist, erythematous with local superficial skin loss; satellite lesions due to candida
Treatment: Keep area dry; topical antifungals (see list in next section), absorbent pwd, 1% hydrocortisone or 0.1% triamcinolone cre bid × 1 or 2 d if inflamed		
Neurodermatitis	Any skin surfaces	Generalized, localized itching
Treatment: Mid- to higher-potency topical corticosteroids (**Table 24**); exclude other causes		
Onychomycosis	Nails	Thickening and discoloration
Treatment: Itraconazole (*Sporanox*)—toenails: 200 mg po qd × 3 mo or 200 mg po bid × 1 wk/mo × 3 mo; fingernails: 200 mg po bid × 1 wk/mo × 2 mo (L); fluconazole (*Diflucan*)—toenails: 150 or 300 mg po/wk × 6–12 mo; fingernails: 150 or 300 mg po/wk × 3–6 mo (L); terbinafine (*Lamisil*)—toenails: 250 mg po qd × 12 wk; fingernails: 250 mg qd × 6 wk. Obtain nail specimens for laboratory culturing to confirm diagnosis before prescribing itraconazole or terbinafine		
Psoriasis	All skin areas, nails (pitting)	Well-defined, erythematous plaques covered with silver scales; severity varies
Treatment: Topical corticosteroids, UV light, PUVA, methotrexate, cyclosporin, etretinate, sulfasalazine; anthralin preparations and tar + 1% to 4% salicylic acid; calcipotriene for nonfacial areas		
Rosacea	Face	Vascular & follicular dilation; mild to moderate
Treatment: Topical metronidazole gel or cre 0.75% bid; oral doxycycline 100 mg qd		
Scabies	Interdigital webs, flexor aspects of wrists, axillary, umbilicus, nipples, genitals	Burrows, erythematous papules or nodules, dry or scaly skin, pruritus
Treatment: Can result in epidemics; treat all contacts and treat environment. Apply topical products from head to toe: Permethrin (*Elimite*) 5% cre q 8–14 h, remove; crotamiton (*Eurax*) 10% cre × 24 h, repeat, then cleansing bath in 48 h; or 1% lindane (*K-well, Scabene*) cre q 8–12 h, remove; oatmeal baths, topical corticosteroids, or emollient creams for symptom relief; ivermectin (*Stromectol*) 200 μg/kg orally; may repeat once in 1 or 2 wk [T: 3, 6]		
Seborrheic dermatitis	Nasal labial folds, eyebrows, hairline, sideburns, posterior auricular and midchest	Greasy, yellow scales with or without erythematous base; common in Parkinson's disease and in debilitated patients
Treatment: Hydrocortisone 1% cre bid or triamcinolone 0.1% oint bid × 2 wk; scalp: shp (selenium sulfide, zinc, or tar); ketoconazole 2% cre for severe conditions when infection from *Pityrosporum orbiculare* is suspected		

Table 23. Dermatologic Conditions Common in Elderly Persons (cont.)		
Condition	**Areas Affected**	**Description**
Skin maceration	Any area constantly in contact with moisture, covered with occlusive dressing or bandage; skin folds, groin, buttocks	Erythema; abraded, excoriated skin; blisters; white and silver patches
Treatment: Eliminate cause of moisture: toileting program for incontinence; condom catheter; indwelling catheter (reserve for most intractable conditions); fecal incontinence collector. Protect skin from moisture: clean gently with mild soap after each incontinent episode; apply moisture barrier (eg, *Vaseline, Proshield, Smooth and Cool, Calmoseptene*) to repel moisture; use disposable briefs that wick moisture from the skin; use linen incontinence pads when disposable briefs accentuate perineal dermatitis.		
Urticaria: Hives	Skin surface	Uniform, red edematous plaques surrounded by white halos
Treatment: Identify cause, oral H$_1$ antihistamines (see **Table 67**), oral glucocorticoids (eg, prednisone 40 mg qd), oral H$_2$ antihistamines, or doxepin (po or topical *Zonalon 5%*) for refractory cases.		
Urticaria: Angioedema	Lips, eyelids, tongue, larynx, GI tract	Larger, deeper than hives
Treatment: Oral H$_1$ antihistamines (see **Table 67**), oral glucocorticoids. Severe reactions: SC epinephrine 0.3 mL of a 1:1000 dilution (*EpiPen*)		
Urticaria: Cholinergic	Skin surface	Round, red papular wheals
Treatment: Oral H$_1$ antihistamines (see **Table 67**) 1 h before exercise. Hot shower may relieve itching.		
Xerosis	All skin surfaces	Dull, rough, flaky, cracked; nummular
Treatment: ↑ Humidity, apply emollient oint (eg, *Aquaphor*) or cre (eg, *Eucerin*) immediately after bathing; oatmeal baths; hydrocortisone 1% oint; avoid excess bathing and bath oils (falls)		

DERMATOLOGIC MEDICATIONS
Topical Antifungals
- Amphotericin B (*Fungizone*) [3% cre, lot, or oint]
- Clotrimazole (*Lotrimin, Mycelex*) [1% cre, lot, sol]
- Econazole nitrate (*Spectazole*) [1% cre]
- Ketoconazole (*Nizoral*) [2% cre or shp]
- Miconazole (eg, *Monistat-Derm*) [2% cre, lot, pwd, spr, tinc]
- Nystatin (*Mycostatin, Nilstat, Nystex*) [100,000 units/g cre, oint, pwd]
- Terbinafine (*Lamisil*–OTC) [1% cre, gel]

Oral Antifungals
- Fluconazole (*Diflucan*) [T: 50, 100, 150, 200; S: 10, 40 mg/mL]
- Itraconazole (*Sporanox*) [C: 100; S: 100 mg/mL]
- Terbinafine (*Lamisil*) [T: 250]

Table 24. Topical Corticosteroids		
Name	Strength & Formulations	Frequency of Application
Lowest Potency		
Dexamethasone phosphate (*Decaderm*)	0.1% cre	qd–qid
Hydrocortisone acetate (*Hytone*)	0.25%, 0.5%, 1%, 2.5% cre, oint	tid–qid
Low Potency		
Alclometasone dipropionate (*Aclovate*)	0.05% cre, oint	bid–tid
Betamethasone valerate (*Valisone*)	0.1% lot	bid–qid
Desonide (*DesOwen, Tridesilon*)	0.05% cre, lot, oint	bid–qid
Fluocinolone acetonide (*Synalar*)	0.025% cre, 0.01% sol	bid–qid
Triamcinolone acetonide (*Aristocort, Kenalog*)	0.1% cre, 0.025% cre, lot, oint	bid–tid
Mid-potency		
Betamethasone dipropionate (*Diprosone*)	0.05% lot	bid–qid
Betamethasone valerate (*Valisone*)	0.1% cre	bid–qid
Clocortolone pivalate (*Cloderm*)	0.1% cre	qd–qid
Desoximetasone (*Topicort*)	0.05% cre	bid
Fluocinolone acetonide (*Synalar*)	0.025% cre, oint	bid–qid
Flurandrenolide (*Cordran*)	0.05% cre, oint, lot	qd–bid
Fluticasone propionate (*Cutivate*)	0.05% cre	bid
Hydrocortisone butyrate (*Locoid*)	0.1% cre	qd–bid
Hydrocortisone valerate (*Westcort*)	0.2% cre, oint	tid–qid
Mometasone furoate (*Elocon*)	0.1% cre, lot	qd
Prednicarbate (*Dermatop*)	0.1% cre, oint	bid
Triamcinolone acetonide (*Aristocort, Kenalog*)	0.1% lot, oint	bid–tid
High Potency		
Amcinonide (*Cyclocort*)	0.1% cre, lot	bid–tid
Betamethasone dipropionate (*Diprosone*)	0.05% cre	bid–qid
Betamethasone valerate (*Valisone*)	0.01% oint	bid–qid
Diflorasone diacetate (*Florone, Maxiflor*)	0.05% cre	bid–qid
Fluocinonide (*Lidex-E*)	0.05% cre	bid–qid
Fluticasone propionate (*Cutivate*)	0.005% oint	bid
Triamcinolone acetonide (*Aristocort, Kenalog*)	0.5% oint	bid–tid
Higher Potency		
Amcinonide (*Cyclocort*)	0.1% oint	bid–tid
Betamethasone dipropionate (*Diprolene AF*)	0.05% augmented cre	bid–qid
Betamethasone dipropionate (*Diprosone*)	0.05% oint	bid–qid
Desoximetasone (*Topicort*)	0.25% cre, oint; 0.05% gel	bid
Diflorasone diacetate (*Florone, Maxiflor*)	0.05% oint	bid–qid
Fluocinonide (*Lidex*)	0.05% cre, oint, gel	bid–qid
Halcinonide (*Halog*)	0.1% cre, oint, sol	qd–tid
Mometasone furoate (*Elocon*)	0.1% oint	qd
Super Potency		
Betamethasone dipropionate (*Diprolene*)	0.05% augmented cre, oint	bid–qid
Clobetasol propionate (*Temovate*)	0.05% cre, oint, sol, gel	bid
Diflorasone diacetate (*Psorcon*)	0.05% optimized oint	qd–tid
Halobetasol propionate (*Ultravate*)	0.05% cre, oint	bid

ENDOCRINE DISORDERS

ADRENAL INSUFFICIENCY
Pharmacologic Therapy
For corticosteroid dose equivalencies, see **Table 25.**

Management
Stress doses of corticosteroids for patients with severe illness, injury, or undergoing surgery: Give hydrocortisone 100 mg IV q 8 h. For less severe stress, double or triple usual oral replacement dose and taper back to baseline as quickly as possible.

Table 25. Corticosteroids					
Drug	Approx Equivalent Dose (mg)	Relative Anti-In-flammatory Potency	Relative Mineral-corticoid	Biologic Half-Life (h)	Formulations
Betamethasone (*Celestone*)	0.6–0.75	20–30	0	36–54	[T: 0.6; S: 0.6 mg/5 mL]
Cortisone (*Cortone*)	25	0.8	2	8–12	[T: 5; S: 50 mg/mL]
Dexamethasone (*Decadron, Dexone, Hexadrol*)	0.75	20–30	0	36–54	[T: 0.25, 0.5, 0.75, 1, 1.5, 2, 4; S: elixir 0.5 mg/5 mL; Inj]
Fludrocortisone (*Florinef*)*	NA	10	4	12–36	[T: 0.1]
Hydrocortisone (*Cortef, Hydrocortone*)	20	1	2	8–12	[T: 5, 10, 20; S: 10 mg/5 mL; Inj]
Methylprednisolone (eg, *Medrol, Solu-Medrol, Depo-Medrol*)	4	5	0	18–36	[T: 2, 4, 8, 16, 24, 32; Inj]
Prednisolone (eg, *Delta-Cortef, Prelone Syr, Pediapred*)	5	4	1	18–36	[S: 5 mg/5 mL; syr 5, 15 mg/5 mL]
Prednisone (*Deltasone, Liquid Pred, Meticorten, Orasone*)	5	4	1	18–36	[T: 1, 2.5, 5, 10, 20, 50; S: 5 mg/5 mL]
Triamcinolone (eg, *Aristocort, Kenacort, Kenalog*)	4	5	0	18–36	[T: 1, 2, 4, 8; S: syr 4 mg/5 mL]

Note: NA = not available.
* Usually given for orthostatic hypotension 0.1 mg qd–tid.

HYPOTHYROIDISM
Common Causes
• Autoimmune (primary thyroid failure)
• Following therapy for hyperthyroidism
• Pituitary or hypothalmic disorders (secondary thyroid failure)
• Medications, especially, amiodarone (rare after first 18 mo of therapy) and lithium

Evaluation
TSH, free T_4

Pharmacologic Therapy
- Thyroxine (T_4, levothyroxine [*Eltroxin, Levo-T, Levothroid, Levoxyl, Synthroid*]). Start 25 μg and increase by 25-μg intervals every 4–6 wk [T: 25, 50, 75, 88, 100, 112, 125, 137, 150, 175, 200, 300 μg].
- Thyroxine and liothyronine (T_3) (*Thyrolar*). Start $\frac{1}{4}$ strength and increase [12.5/3.1 ($\frac{1}{4}$ strength), 25/6.25 ($\frac{1}{2}$ strength), 50/12.5, 100/25, 150/37.5 μg].
- For myxedema coma: Load 400 μg IV or 100 μg q 6–8 h for 1 d, then 100 μg/d for 4 d; then start usual replacement regimen.
- To convert thyroid USP to thyroxine: 60 mg USP = 50 μg thyroxine.
- If patients are npo and must receive IV thyroxine, dose should be half usual po dose.

Monitoring
In primary hypothyroidism, the goal of therapy is to maintain plasma TSH within the normal range. Further adjustments are made every 6–12 wk (12- to 25-μg increments) on basis of TSH levels until TSH is in normal range. Monitor TSH level every 6–12 mo (ATA) in patients on chronic thyroid replacement therapy. Following dose adjustment, recheck TSH in 6–12 wk.

HYPERTHYROIDISM
Common Causes
- Graves' disease
- Toxic nodule
- Toxic multinodular goiter
- Medications, esp. amiodarone (can occur any time during therapy) and lithium

Evaluation
TSH, free T_4. When indicated, T_3, thyroid autoantibodies, radioactive iodine uptake.

Pharmacologic Therapy
- Radioactive iodine ablation is usual treatment of choice, but surgery or medical therapy (see Monitoring above) are options.
- Propylthiouracil (PTU): Start 100 po tid, then adjust up to 200 po tid as needed [T: 50].
- Methimazole (*Tapazole*): Start 5–20 mg po tid, then adjust [T: 5, 10].
- Adjunctive therapy with β-blockers (see Table 16) or calcium antagonists (see **Table 16**) may provide symptomatic improvement.

DIABETES MELLITUS
Definition and Classification (ADA)
Diabetes mellitus is a group of metabolic diseases characterized by hyperglycemia resulting from defects in insulin secretion, insulin action, or both.
Type 1: Caused by an absolute deficiency of insulin secretion.
Type 2: Caused by a combination of resistance to insulin action and an inadequate compensatory insulin secretory response.

Criteria for Diagnosis: One or more of the following:
- Symptoms of diabetes (eg, polyuria, polydipsia, unexplained weight loss) plus casual plasma glucose concentration $\geq$ 200 mg/dL
- Fasting (no caloric intake for $\geq$ 8 h) plasma glucose $\geq$ 126 mg/dL
- 2 h Plasma glucose $\geq$ 200 mg/dL during an oral glucose tolerance test (OGTT)
Diagnosis should be confirmed by reevaluating on a subsequent day.
Impaired Fasting Glucose: Defined as fasting plasma glucose $\geq$ 110 and < 126 mg/dL
Impaired Glucose Tolerance: Abnormal casual plasma glucose concentration or response to OGTT but not meeting diagnostic criteria for diabetes

Management
Goals of Treatment (ADA): Average preprandial capillary blood glucose 80–120 mg/dL, average bedtime capillary blood glucose 100–140 mg/dL, and HbA$_{1c}$ < 7%
Nonpharmacologic Interventions:
- Individualized nutrition therapy (see p 90)
- Life style (eg, regular exercise, alcohol and smoking cessation)
- Patient and family education for self-management
- Self-monitoring of blood glucose
- High-fiber diet (25 g insoluble and 25 g soluble/d)

Pharmacologic Interventions for Type 2: Stepped therapy:
1. Monotherapy with a 2nd-generation sulfonylurea agent, α-glucosidase inhibitor, metformin, or thiazolidinedione (see **Table 26**)
2. Combination therapy with 2 or more agents with different actions
3. Add insulin hs or switch to insulin bid (see **Table 27**)
Manage hypertension (BP goal < 130/80 mm Hg; also see p 29) and lipid disorders (p 28; treat as CHD risk equivalent), as appropriate. ACE inhibitor or angiotensin II receptor blocker (ARB) if albuminuria, hypertension, or another cardiovascular risk factor. If ACE inhibitor or ARB not tolerated; consider nondihydropyridine calcium channel blocker. Daily ASA 81–325 mg.

Table 26. Oral Agents for Treating Diabetes Mellitus			
Drug	**Dosage**	**Formulations**	**Comments (Metabolism)**
2nd-Generation Sulfonylureas			Stimulate insulin secretion
Glimepiride (*Amaryl*)	4–8 mg once, begin 1–2 mg	[T: 1, 2, 4]	Numerous drug interactions, long-acting (L, K)
Glipizide (generic or *Glucotrol*)	2.5–40 mg once or divided	[T: 5, 10]	Short-acting (L, K)
(*Glucotrol XL*)	5–20 mg once	[T: ER 2.5, 5, 10]	Long-acting (L, K)
Glyburide (generic or *Diaβeta, Micronase*)	1.25–20 mg once or divided	[T: 1.25, 2.5, 5]	Long-acting, risk of hypoglycemia (L, K)
Micronized glyburide (*Glynase*)	1.5–12 mg once	[T: 1.5, 3, 4.5, 6]	(L, K)
α-Glucosidase Inhibitors			Delay glucose absorption
Acarbose (*Precose*)	50–100 mg tid, just before meals, start with 25 mg	[T: 25, 50, 100]	GI side effects common, avoid if creatinine > 2 mg/dL, monitor LFTs (gut, K)

(*continues*)

Table 26. Oral Agents for Treating Diabetes Mellitus (cont.)			
Drug	**Dosage**	**Formulations**	**Comments (Metabolism)**
Miglitol (*Glyset*)	25–100 mg tid, with 1st bite of meal; start with 25 mg qd	[T: 25, 50, 100]	Same as acarbose but no need to monitor LFTs (L, K)
Biguanides			Insulin sensitizers
Metformin (*Glucophage*) (*Glucophage XR*)	500–2550 divided 1500–2000 qd	[T: 500, 850, 1000] [T: ER 500]	Avoid in patients > 80 yr, $Cr > 1.5$ in men, $Cr > 1.4$ in women, CHF, COPD, ↑ LFTs (K)
Meglitinides			Increase insulin secretion
Nateglinide (*Starlix*)	60–120 mg tid	[T: 60, 120]	Give 30 min before meals
Repaglinide (*Prandin*)	0.5 mg bid–qid if HbA$_{1c}$ < 8% or previously untreated 1–2 mg bid–qid if HbA$_{1c}$ ≥ 8% or previously treated	[T: 0.5, 1, 2]	Give 30 min before meals, adjust dose at wkly intervals; potential for drug interactions, caution in liver, renal insufficiency (L)
Thiazolidinediones			Insulin resistance reducers; ↑ risk of CHF; avoid if NYHA Class III or IV cardiac status; D/C if any decline in cardiac status
Pioglitazone (*Actos*)	15 or 30 mg qd; max 45 mg/d as monotherapy, 30 mg/d in combination therapy	[T: 15, 30, 45]	Check LFTs at start, q 2 mo during 1st yr, then periodically; avoid if clinical evidence of liver disease or if serum ALT levels > 2.5 upper limit of normal (L, K)
Rosiglitazone (*Avandia*)	4 mg qd–bid	[T: 2, 4, 8]	Check LFTs at start, q 2 mo during 1st yr, then periodically; avoid if clinical evidence of liver disease or if serum ALT levels > 2.5 upper limit of normal (L, K)
Combinations			
Glipizide & metformin (*Metaglip*)	2.5/250 once; 20/2000 in 2 divided doses	[T: 2.5/250, 2.5/500, 5/500]	Avoid in patients > 80 yr, $Cr > 1.5$ in men, $Cr > 1.4$ in women; see individual drugs (L, K)
Glyburide & metformin (*Glucovance*)	1.25/250 mg initially if previously untreated; 2.5/500 mg or 5/500 mg bid with meals; maximum 20/2000/d	[T: 1.25/250, 2.5/500, 5/500]	Starting dose should not exceed the total daily dose of either drug; see also individual drugs
Rosiglitizone & metformin (*Avandamet*)	4/1000–8/2000 in 2 divided doses	[T: 1/500, 2/500, 4/500]	Avoid in patients > 80 yr, $Cr > 1.5$ in men, $Cr > 1.4$ in women; see individual drugs (L, K)

Table 27. Insulin Preparations			
Preparations	Onset	Peak	Duration
Insulin lispro (*Humalog*)	15 min	0.5–1.5 h	6–8 h
Insulin (eg, *Humulin, Novolin*)*			
Regular	0.5–1 h	2–3 h	8–12 h
NPH	1–1.5 h	4–12 h	24 h
Insulin aspart (*NovoLog*)	30 min	1–3 h	3–5 h
Long-acting (*Ultralente*)	4–8 h	16–18 h	> 36 h
Insulin glargine (*Lantus*)**	1–2 h	—	24 h
Insulin, zinc (*Lente*)	1–2.5 h	8–12 h	18–24 h
Isophane insulin & regular insulin inj. (*Novolin 70/30*)	0.5 h	2–12 h	24 h

* Also available as mixtures of NPH and regular in 50:50 proportions.
** To convert from NPH dosing, give same number of units at bedtime. For patients taking NPH bid, decrease the total daily units by 20%, give at bedtime, and titrate on basis of response.

Monitoring (ADA)
- Weight, BP, and foot examination, including monofilament, palpation, and inspection, each visit
- HbA$_{1c}$ twice/yr in patients with stable glycemic control; quarterly, if poor control
- Annual comprehensive dilated eye and visual examinations by an ophthalmologist or optometrist who is experienced in management of diabetic retinopathy
- Lipid profiles every 1–2 yr depending on whether values are in normal range
- Annual (unless microalbuminuria has previously been demonstrated) test for microalbuminuria by measuring albumin-to-creatinine ratio in a random spot collection, timed collection, or 24-h collection

FALLS

DEFINITION
An event that results in a person's inadvertently coming to rest on the ground or lower level with or without loss of consciousness or injury. Excludes falls from major intrinsic event (seizure, stroke, syncope) or overwhelming environmental hazard.

ETIOLOGY
Typically multifactorial. Composed of intrinsic (eg, poor balance, weakness, chronic illness, visual or cognitive impairment), extrinsic (eg, polypharmacy), and environmental (eg, poor lighting, no safety equipment, loose carpets) factors. Commonly a nonspecific sign for one of many acute illnesses in older persons.

EVALUATION
Exclude acute illness or underlying systemic or metabolic process (eg, infection, electrolyte imbalance as indicated by history, examination, and laboratory studies). See **Figure 3** for recommended assessment and management.

History
- Circumstances of fall (eg, activity at time of fall, location, time)
- Associated symptoms (eg, lightheadedness, vertigo, syncope, weakness, confusion, palpitations)
- Relevant comorbid conditions (eg, prior stroke, parkinsonism, cardiac disease, seizure disorder, depression, anxiety, anemia, sensory deficit, glaucoma, cataracts, osteoporosis, cognitive impairment)
- Previous falls
- Medication review, including OTC medications and alcohol use; note recent changes in medications; note drugs that have hypotensive or psychoactive effects (see page 60)

Physical
Look for:
- Vital signs: postural pulse and BP changes, fever, hypothermia
- Head and neck: visual impairment (especially poor acuity, reduced contrast sensitivity, decreased visual fields, cataracts), motion-induced imbalance (Dix-Hallpike test), bruit, nystagmus
- Musculoskeletal: arthritic changes, motion or joint limitations (especially lower extremity joint function), postural instability, skeletal deformities, podiatric problems
- Neurologic: slower reflexes, altered proprioception, altered mental status, focal deficits, peripheral neuropathy, gait or balance disorders, muscle weakness (especially leg), instability, tremor, rigidity
- Cardiovascular: heart arrhythmias, cardiac valve dysfunction
- Other: fever; hypothermia

Figure 3. Assessment and Management of Falls

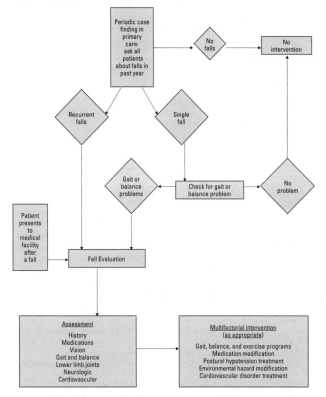

Source: American Geriatrics Society, British Geriatrics Society, and American Academy of Orthopaedic Surgeons Panel on Falls Prevention. Guideline for the prevention of falls in older persons. *J Amer Geristr Soc.* **2001; 49(5):666.** Reprinted with permission.

Functional Assessment
- Functional gait: observe patient rising from chair, walking (stride, length, velocity, symmetry), turning, sitting (Timed Get Up and Go test; see also POMA, p 174.)
- Balance: Side-by-side, semi-tandem, and full tandem stance; Functional Reach test (see also POMA, p 174.)
- Mobility: observe the patient's use of assistive device (cane, walker, or personal assistance), extent of ambulation, restraint use, footwear evaluation

Ask about person's ability to complete activities of daily living: bathing, dressing, transferring, continence.

Medications Associated with Increased Fall Risk
- Antipsychotics (especially phenothiazines)
- Sedatives, hypnotics (including benzodiazepines)
- Antihypertensives (including diuretics, vasodilators)
- Antidepressants (including MAOIs, SSRIs, TCAs)
- Antiarrhythmics (including digoxin)
- Antihistamines
- Analgesics (including NSAIDs, opioids)

PREVENTION
Goal is to minimize risk of falling without compromising mobility and functional independence.
- Fall risk assessment should be part of every routine primary health care visit (at least annually).
- Assess for risk factors using a multidisciplinary approach, if appropriate, including medical and occupational therapy.
- Target interventions to risk factors (see **Table 28**). Correction of postural hypotension, review and modification of medications, and interventions to improve balance, transfers, and gait are priority.
- Choose fall prevention programs that include more than one intervention. A structured, interdisciplinary approach should be used.
  - Establish tailored exercise programs targeted at older people with mild deficits in strength, balance, lower extremity strength, and range of motion.
  - Tai Chi classes should be offered to older people living in the community.
  - Counsel older patients on measures to reduce the risk of falling, including exercise, safety-related skills and behaviors, and environmental hazard reduction.
  - Offer hip protectors to all residents of nursing homes and others at high risk—available via http://www.hipprotector.com or http://www.hipsaver.com.
- Focus on most common risk factors: Muscle weakness, history of falls, gait deficit, balance deficit, use of assistive devices, visual deficit, arthritis, impaired ADLs, depression, cognitive impairment, age > 80 yr.

Table 28. Preventing Falls: Selected Risk Factors and Suggested Interventions	
Factors	**Suggested Interventions**
Medication-related factors	
Use of benzodiazepines, sedative-hypnotics, or antipsychotic	Consider agents with less risk for falls (eg, atypical antipsychotics such as olanzapine, risperidone, or quetiapine)
	Taper and D/C medications, as possible
	Address sleep problems with nonpharmacologic interventions (see p 155)
	Educate regarding use of medications and monitoring for side effects
Recent change in dose *or* number of prescriptions medications *or* use of ≥ 4 prescription medications *or* use of other medications associated with fall risk	Review medication profile and modify, as possible
	Monitor response to medications and to dose changes
Mobility-related factors	
Presence of environmental hazards (eg, improper bed height, cluttered walking surfaces, lack of railings, poor lighting)	Improve lighting
	Remove floor barriers (eg, loose carpeting)
	Replace existing furniture with safer furniture (eg, correct height, more stable)
	Install support structures (eg, railings, grab bars)
Impaired gait, balance, or transfer skills	Gait training
	Balance or strengthening exercises
	Provide training in transfer skills
	Prescribe appropriate assistive devices
	Recommend protective hip padding
	Environmental changes (eg, grab bars, raised toilet seats)
Impaired leg or arm strength or range of motion	Prescribe strengthening exercises (eg, use of resistive rubber bands, putty)
	Prescribe resistance training 2–3 wk to 10 repetitions with full range of motion, then increase resistance
	Tai Chi
	Physical therapy
Medical factors	
Parkinson's disease, osteoarthritis, other conditions associated with increased falls	Optimize medical therapy
	Monitor for disease progression and impact on mobility and impairments
	Determine need for assistive devices
Postural hypotension: drop in SBP > 20 mm Hg or to ≤ 90 mm Hg on standing	Review medications potentially contributing and adjust dosing or switch to less hypotensive agents
	Educate on activities to decrease effect (eg, slow rising, ankle pumps, hand clenching, elevation of head of bed)
	Prescribe pressure stockings (eg, Jobst)
	Consider medication to increase pressure:
	-fludrocortisone (*Florinef*) 0.1 mg qd–tid [T: 0.1]
	-midodrine (*ProAmatine*) 2.5–5 mg tid [T: 2.5, 5]
	-caffeinated coffee (1 cup) or caffeine 100 mg with meals

GASTROINTESTINAL DISEASES

DYSPHAGIA
See p 123.

GASTROESOPHAGEAL REFLUX DISEASE (GERD)

Definition
The retrograde movement of the gastric contents in the esophagus due to incompetent lower esophageal sphincter, transient relaxations of the sphincter, or compromise of other antireflux mechanisms.

Evaluation and Assessment
Empiric treatment is appropriate when hx is typical for uncomplicated GERD.
- Endoscopy (if symptoms persist despite initial management, atypical presentation, or longstanding symptoms)
- 24-h pH monitoring

Symptoms Suggesting Complicated GERD and Need For Evaluation
- Dysphagia
- Bleeding
- Weight loss
- Choking (acid causing cough, SOB, or hoarseness)
- Chest pain

Management
Nonpharmacologic:
- Antacids
- Avoid alcohol and fatty foods
- Avoid lying down 3 h after eating
- Avoid tight-fitting clothes
- Change diet (avoid pepper, spearmint, chocolate, spicy or acidic foods)
- Drink 6–8 oz water with all medications
- Elevate head of the bed (6–8 in)
- Lose weight (if overweight)
- Stop drugs that may promote reflux
- Stop smoking
- Consider surgery

Pharmacologic:

Table 29. Pharmacologic Management of GERD		
Drug	**Initial Oral Dosage**	**Formulations (Excretion)**
Proton-Pump Inhibitors		
Esomeprazole (*Nexium*)	20 mg qd × 4 wk	[C: ER 20, 40] (L)
Lansoprazole (*Prevacid*)	15 mg qd × 8 wk	[C: ER 15, 30; granules for susp: 15, 30/packet] (L)
Omeprazole (*Prilosec*)	20 mg qd × 4–8 wk	[C: ER 10, 20, 40] (L)
Pantoprazole (*Protonix*)	40 mg qd × 8 wk	[T: enteric-coated, 20, 40; Inj]
Rabeprazole (*Aciphex*)	20 mg qd × 8 wk; 20 mg qd maintenance, if needed	[T: enteric-coated ER 20] (L)
H₂ Antagonists (for less severe GERD)		
Cimetidine (*Tagamet*)	400 or 800 mg bid	[S: 200 mg/20 mL, 300 mg/5 mL with alcohol 2.8%; T: 100, 200,* 300, 400, 800; Inj] (K, L)

Table 29. Pharmacologic Management of GERD (cont.)		
Drug	Initial Oral Dosage	Formulations (Excretion)
Famotidine (*Pepcid*)	20 mg bid × 6 wk	[S: oral sus 40 mg/5 mL; T: film-coated 10,*. 20, 40, oral disintegrating 20, 40; C (gel): 10*; ChT: 10*;Inj] (K)
Nizatidine (*Axid*)	150 mg bid	[C: 150, 300; T: 75] (K)
Ranitidine (*Zantac*)	150 mg bid	[Pk: gran, effervescent (EFFERdose) 150 mg; S: syr 15 mg/mL; T: 75,* 150, 300; T: effervescent (EFFERdose) 150; Inj] (K, F)
Mucosal Protective Agent		
Sucralfate (*Carafate*)	1 g qid, 1h ac and hs	[S: oral sus 1 g/10 mL; T: 1 g] (F, K)
Prokinetic Agents		
Bethanechol (*Urecholine*)	25 mg qid	[T: 5, 10, 25, 50] (unknown)
Metoclopramide† (*Reglan*)	5 mg qid, ac, and hs	[S: syr, sugar-free 5 mg/5 mL, conc 10 mg/mL; T: 5, 10; Inj] (K, F)

* OTC strength.
† Risk of extrapyramidal symptoms high in persons aged > 65 yr.
Source: Data from DeVault KR, Castell DO. Updated guidelines for the diagnosis and treatment of gastroesophageal reflux disease. *Am J Gastroenterol.* 1999;94:1430–1442.

PEPTIC ULCER DISEASE
Causes
Helicobacter pylori is the major cause. NSAIDs are the second most common cause.

Diagnosis of *H pylori*
- Endoscopic examination
- Serology
- Urea breath test

Initial Treatment Options
- Empiric anti-ulcer treatment for 6 wk
- Definitive diagnostic evaluation by endoscopy
- Noninvasive testing for *H pylori* and treatment with antibiotics for (+) patients (see **Table 30** for regimens)
- Review patient's chronic medications for drug interactions before selecting regimen; many potential drug interactions and adverse drug reactions.

Table 30. FDA-Approved Treatments for *H. pylori*–Induced Ulcerations (all oral routes)
Lansoprazole 30 mg bid + amoxicillin 1 g bid + clarithromycin 500 mg tid × 10 (or 14) d
or Omeprazole 20 mg bid + clarithromycin 500 mg bid + amoxicillin 1 g bid × 10 d
or Lansoprazole 30 mg bid + clarithromycin 500 mg bid + amoxicillin 1 g bid × 10 d (*Prevpac*)
or Omeprazole 40 mg qd + clarithromycin 500 mg tid × 2 wk, then omeprazole 20 mg qd × 2 wk
or Lansoprazole 30 mg tid + amoxicillin 1 g bid × 2 wk (only for person allergic or intolerant to clarithromycin)

(*continues*)

or Ranitidine bismuth citrate (RBC) 400 mg bid + clarithromycin 500 mg tid × 2 wk, then RBC 400 mg bid × 2 wk

or RBC 400 mg bid + clarithromycin 500 mg bid × 2 wk, then RBC 400 mg bid × 2 wk

or Bismuth subsalicylate (*Pepto-Bismol*) 525 mg qid (pc and hs) + metronidazole 250 mg qid + tetracycline 500 mg qid × 2 wk (*Helidac*) + H₂ receptor antagonist therapy as directed × 4 wk

Source: http://www.cdc.gov/ulcer/md.htm.
For additional, non-FDA approved regimens, see Howden CW, Hunt RH. Guidelines for the management of *Helicobacter pylori* infection. *Am J Gastroenterol* 1998;93:2330–2338, or http://www.acg.gi.org.

Medications
Bismuth subsalicylate (*Pepto-Bismol*) [T: 324; ChT: 262; S: sus 262 mg/15 mL, 525 mg/15 mL]
Antibiotics: (for complete information, see **Table 45**)
Amoxicillin (*Amoxil*) [C: 250, 500; ChT: 125, 250; S: oral sus 125 mg/5 mL, 250 mg/5 mL]
Clarithromycin (*Biaxin*) [T: film-coated 250, 500; S: oral sus 125 mg/5 mL, 250 mg/5 mL]
Metronidazole (*Flagyl*) [T: 250, 500, 750; C: 375]
Tetracycline (*Achromycin, Sumycin*) [T: 250, 500; S: oral sus 125 mg/5 mL]
Proton-Pump Inhibitors: See **Table 29**.
H₂ Antagonist Combination:
Ranitidine bismuth citrate [ranitidine 162 mg, trivalent bismuth 128 mg, and citrate 110 mg] (*Tritec*) [T: 400]

STRESS-ULCER PREVENTION IN HOSPITALIZED OLDER PERSONS
Risk Factors (in order of prevalence in older persons)
• Hx of GI ulceration or bleed in the past year
• Sepsis
• Multiple organ failure
• Hypotension
• Respiratory failure requiring mechanical ventilation > 48 h
• Renal failure
• Major trauma, shock, or head injury
• Coagulopathy (platelets < 50,000/μL, INR > 1.5, or PTT > 2 × control)
• Burns over > 25% of body surface area
• Hepatic failure
• Intracranial hypertension
• Spinal cord injury
• Tetraplegia
Prophylaxis
• H₂ antagonists (see **Table 29**)
• Proton-pump inhibitors (see **Table 29**)
• Sucralfate (see **Table 29**)
• Antacids
• Enteral feedings

Key points
- Prophylaxis has not been shown to reduce mortality
- No one regimen has shown superior efficacy
- Choice of regimen depends on access to and function of GI tract and presence of continuous nasogastric suction

CONSTIPATION
Definition
Infrequent, incomplete, or painful evacuation of feces.

Drugs That Constipate
- Analgesics—opiates
- Antacids with aluminum or calcium
- Anticholinergic drugs
- Antidepressants, lithium
- Antihypertensives
- Antipsychotics
- Barium sulfate
- Bismuth
- Calcium channel blockers
- Diuretics
- Iron

Conditions That Constipate
- Colon tumor or mechanical obstruction
- Dehydration
- Depression
- Diabetes mellitus
- Hypercalcemia
- Hypokalemia
- Hypothyroidism
- Immobility
- Low intake of fiber
- Panhypopituitarism
- Parkinson's disease
- Spinal cord injury
- Stroke
- Uremia

Management of Chronic Constipation
Step 1. Stop all constipating medications, when possible.
Step 2. Increase dietary bran to 6–25 g/d and increase fluid intake to $\geq$ 1500 mL/d and increase physical activity.
Step 3. Add bran supplements, provided fluid intake is $\geq$ 1500 mL/d.
Step 4. Add 70% sorbitol solution (15–30 mL qd or bid, max 150 mL/d).
Step 5. Add stimulant laxative (eg, senna, bisacodyl), 2–3 times/wk. (Alternative: Saline laxative, but avoid in renal insufficiency.)
Step 6. Use tap water enema or saline enema 2 times/wk.
Step 7. Use oil-retention enema for refractory constipation.

Table 31. Medications That May Relieve Constipation			
Medication	**Onset of Action**	**Starting Dosage**	**Site and Mechanism of Action**
Bisacodyl tablet (*Dulcolax*)	6–10 h	5–15 mg × 1	Colon
Bisacodyl suppository (*Dulcolax*)	0.25–1 h	10 mg × 1	Colon
Docusate (*Colace*)	24–72 h	100 mg qd–qid	Small and large intestine; detergent activity; facilitates admixture of fat and water to soften stool

(*continues*)

Table 31. Medications That May Relieve Constipation (cont.)			
Medication	**Onset of Action**	**Starting Dosage**	**Site and Mechanism of Action**
Lactulose (*Cephulac*)*	24–48 h	15–30 mL qd–bid	Colon; osmotic effect
Magnesium citrate (*Citroma*)	0.5–3 h	120–240 mL × 1	Small and large intestine; attracts, retains water in intestinal lumen
Magnesium hydroxide (*Milk of Magnesia*)	30 min–3 h	30 mL qd–bid	Osmotic effect and increased peristalsis in colon
Methylcellulose psyllium (*Metamucil*)	12–24 h (up to 72 h)	1–2 rounded tsp or packets qd–tid with water or juice	Small and large intestine; holds water in stool; mechanical distention
Polyethylene glycol (*MiraLax*)	48–96 h	17 g pwd qd (~1 tablespoon) dissolved in 8 oz water	GI tract; osmotic effect
Sodium phosphate/ biphosphate emollient enema (*Fleet*)	2–15 min	1 4.5-oz enema × 1, repeat prn	Colon
Senna (*Senoket*)	6–10 h	2 tabs or 1 tsp qhs	Colon; direct action on intestine; stimulates myenteric plexus; alters water and electrolyte secerction
Sorbitol 70%	24–48 h	15–30 mL qd–bid	Colon; delivers osmotically active molecules to colon

* By prescription only.

NAUSEA AND VOMITING
Causes
- CNS disorders (eg, motion sickness, intracranial lesions)
- Drugs (eg, chemotherapy, NSAIDs, narcotic analgesics, antibiotics, digoxin)
- GI disorders (eg, mechanical obstruction; inflammation of stomach, intestine, or gallbladder; pseudo-obstruction, motility disorders, dyspepsia, diabetic gastroparesis)
- Infections (eg, viral or bacterial gastroenteritis, hepatitis, otitis, meningitis)
- Metabolic conditions (eg, uremia, acidosis, hyperparathyroidism, adrenal insufficiency)
- Psychiatric disorders

Evaluation
- If patient is not seriously ill or dehydrated, can probably wait 24–48 h to see if symptoms resolve spontaneously.
- If patient is seriously ill, dehydrated, or has other signs of acute illness, hospitalize for further evaluation.
- If symptoms persist, evaluate according to suspected causes.

Pharmacologic Management

Drugs that are useful in the management of nausea and vomiting are listed in **Table 32**.

Table 32. Selected Antiemetics		
Drug	**Formulations**	**Dosages (Metabolism)**
Dimenhydrinate* (*Dramamine*)	[Inj; S: 12.5 mg/4 mL, 16.62 mg/5 mL; T: 50; ChT: 50]	Oral, IM IV; 50–100 mg q 4–6 h, not to exceed 400 mg/d (L)
Meclizine* (*Antivert*)	[C: 25, 30; T: 12.5, 25, 50; ChT: 25; T: film-coated 25]	Motion sickness: 12.5–25 mg 1 h before travel, repeat dose q 12–24 h if needed; doses up to 50 mg may be needed; vertigo: 25–100 mg/d in divided doses (L)
Metoclopramide (*Reglan*)	[Inj; S: oral conc 10 mg/mL, syr, sugar-free, 5 mg/5 mL; T: 5, 10]	Chemotherapy-induced emesis, IV: 1–2 mg/kg 30 min before chemotherapy and q 2–4 to q 4–6 h; postoperative nausea and vomiting: IM 5–10 mg near the end of surgery (K)
Prochlorperazine (*Compazine*)	[C: ER: 10, 15, 30; Inj; Sp: 2.5, 5, 25; S: syr 5 mg/5 mL; T: 5, 10, 25]	Oral or IM: 5–10 mg 3–4 times/d, usual maximum, 40 mg/d; IV: 2.5–10 mg; maximum 10 mg/dose or 40 mg/d; may repeat dose q 3–4 h as needed; rectal: 25 mg bid (L)

* Available OTC.
Note: All have potential CNS toxicity.

DIARRHEA
Causes
- Drugs (eg, antibiotics [see **Table 45**], laxatives, colchicine)
- Fecal impaction
- GI disorders (eg, irritable bowel syndrome, malabsorption, inflammatory bowel disease)
- Infections (eg, viral, bacterial, parasitic)
- Lactose intolerance

Evaluation
- If patient is not seriously ill or dehydrated and there is no blood in the stool, can probably wait 48 h to see if symptoms resolve spontaneously.
- If patient is seriously ill, dehydrated, or has other signs of acute illness, hospitalize for further evaluation.
- If diarrhea persists, evaluate on the basis of the most likely causes.

Pharmacologic Management

Drugs that are useful in the management of diarrhea are listed in **Table 33**.

Table 33. Antidiarrheals		
Drug	**Dosage (Metabolism)**	**Formulations**
Attapulgite* (*Kaopectate*)	1200–1500 mg after each loose bowel movement or q 2 h; 15–30 mL up to 9 × /d, up to 9000 mg/24 h (not absorbed)	[S: oral conc 600, 750 mg/ 15 mL; T: 750; ChT: 300, 600]
Bismuth subsalicylate* (*Pepto-Bismol*)	2 tablets or 30 mL q 30 min to 1 h as needed up to 8 doses/ 24 h	[S: 262 mg/15 mL, 525 mg/ 15 mL; T: 324; ChT: 262]
Diphenoxylate with atropine (*Lomotil*)†	15–20 mg/d of diphenoxylate in 3–4 divided doses; maintenance 5–15 mg/d in 2–3 divided doses (L)	[S: oral, diphenoxylate hydrochloride 2.5 mg + atropine sulfate 0.025 mg/5 mL; T: diphenoxylate hydrochloride 2.5 mg and atropine sulfate 0.025 mg]
Loperamide* (*Imodium A-D*)	Initial: 4 mg (2 capsules), followed by 2 mg after each loose stool, up to 16 mg/d (8 capsules) (L)	[Caplet, 2; C: 2; T: 2; S: oral, 1 mg/5 mL]

* Available OTC.
† Anticholinergic, potentially CNS toxic.

HEARING IMPAIRMENT

DEFINITION
The most common sensory impairment in old age. To quantify hearing ability, the necessary intensity (decibel = dB) and frequency (Hertz) of the perceived pure-tone signal must be described.

EVALUATION
Screening
- Note problems during conversation
- Ask about hearing dysfunction
- Use a standardized questionnaire (see p 173)
- Test with handheld audioscope
- Use whisper test—stand behind patient 2 ft from ear, cover untested ear, fully exhale, whisper an easily answered question
- Refer patients who screen positive for audiologic evaluation

Audiometry
- Documents the dB loss across frequencies
- Determines the pattern of loss (see Classification, below)
- Determines if loss is unilateral or bilateral **Note:** If speech discrimination is less than 50%, results with hearing aids may be poor

Aggravating Factors
- Sensorineural loss—medication ototoxicity (eg, aminoglycosides, loop diuretics, cisplatin), cerumen impaction (see page 70)
- Conductive loss—cerumen impaction, external otitis

CLASSIFICATION
Sensorineural Hearing Loss
Due to cochlear or retrocochlear pathology; both air and bone conduction thresholds are increased; causes: aging, eighth nerve damage from syphilis, viral meningitis, trauma, vascular events to eighth nerve or cortical tracts, acoustic neuroma, Ménière's disease.

Conductive Hearing Loss
Occurs when sound transmission to inner ear is impaired; bone conduction better than air conduction; causes include: external or middle ear disorders, including otosclerosis; rheumatoid arthritis; Paget's disease.

Central Auditory Processing Disorder
Loss of speech discrimination in excess of that from loss in hearing sensitivity; involves the CNS; occurs in dementia and infrequently with presbycusis.

Presbycusis (Old-Age Hearing Loss, a Subtype of Sensorineural Loss):
- Mainly high-frequency loss
- Impaired speech discrimination
- Recruitment (an increase in sensation of loudness)
- Both bone and air conduction affected

Figure 4. Degrees of Hearing Loss in Presbycusis, by Audiometry (see Table 34)

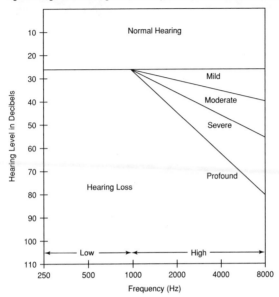

MANAGEMENT
Remove Ear Wax
Fill ear canal with 5–10 gtt water and cover with cotton bid × 4d or more. Liquid must stay in contact with ear for at least 15 min. Hearing may worsen as cerumen expands. Water is as effective as commercial preparations (eg, *Debrox, Cerumenex, Colace*).

Table 34. Effects and Rehabilitation of Hearing Loss, by Level of Loss		
Level of Loss	**Difficulty Understanding**	**Need for Hearing Aid**
0–24 dB	None	None
25–40 dB (mild)	Normal speech	In specific situations
41–55 dB (moderate)	Loud speech	Frequent
56–80 dB (severe)	Anything but amplified speech	For all communication
81 dB or more (profound)	Even amplified speech	Plus speech reading, aural rehabilitation, or sign language

Source: Data in part from *A Report on Hearing Aids: User Perspectives and Concerns.* Washington, DC: American Association of Retired Persons; 1993:2.

Hearing Devices

Hearing Aids: Appropriate for most hearing-impaired persons; enhance select frequencies; should be individualized for each ear. Amplification in both ears (binaural) achieves best speech understanding; unilateral aid may be appropriate if asymmetrical speech discrimination, if hearing aid care is challenging, or because of cost.

Implantable Hearing Devices: Are FDA approved for adults with moderate to severe sensorineural hearing loss. Expensive.

Assistive Listening Devices: Microphone placed close to sound source transmits to headphones or earpiece. Transmission is by wire or wireless (FM or infrared); these systems increase signal-to-noise ratio, which is useful for persons with central auditory processing disorder.

Telephone Device for the Deaf (TDD): Receiver is a keyboard that allows the hearing-impaired person to respond.

Tips for Communication with Hearing-Impaired Persons

- Stand 2–3 ft away
- Have the person's attention
- Have the person seated in front of a wall, which will help reflect sound
- Use lower-pitched voice
- Speak slowly and distinctly; don't shout
- Rephrase rather than repeat
- Pause at the end of phrases or ideas

HEMATOLOGY AND ONCOLOGY

ANEMIA
Evaluation
- Some decrease in hemoglobin with age is normal.
- Evaluate persons > 65 when Hb < 12 in men and when Hb < 11.5 in women.
- Evaluate if Hb falls > 1 g/dL in 1 yr.
- Check reticulocyte count for hypo- or hyperregenerative disorder (see **Table 35**).
- Obtain bone marrow aspirate and biopsy if causes not clear.

Treatment

Table 35. Diagnosis and Management of Anemia

Anemia Type	Findings & Considerations	Management
Hyporegenerative		
Chronic disorders	↓ Reticulocyte count Normocytic or microcytic RBCs Chronic underlying disease Iron studies, erythropoietin level	Treat underlying disorder; low erythropoietin level predicts response to: Erythropoietin 50–100 U/kg q wk; increase dose to 150 U/kg if no response in 2–3 wk. Indicated in chronic renal failure, during cancer therapy, possibly CHF
Iron deficiency	Serum ferritin ≤ 50 μg/L with transferrin saturation ≤ 0.08 Serum ferritin ≤ 20 μg/L	Correct cause of blood loss Oral iron supplements: ferrous sulfate 325 mg po qd; parenteral iron* if iron absorption poor or not tolerated
B$_{12}$ deficiency	Macrocytosis, giant and multi-lobar neutrophils, ↓ platelets; serum B$_{12}$, folate, and TSH; methylmalonic in selected patients**	B$_{12}$ 1000 μg/wk × 5 wk, then 100 μg IM/mo or 1000 μg po daily for life Potassium for the 1st wk and iron supplement if anemia is severe
Aplastic anemia	Pancytopenia; bone marrow aspirate and biopsy; tartrate-resistant acid phosphatase; bone marrow chromosomal analysis	Consult hematology for diagnosis and differential diagnosis of myelodysplastic disorders
Hyperregenerative		
Hemolytic anemia	↑ Reticulocyte count, ↑ indirect bilirubin, Coombs' test often positive; associated with drug effects, chronic lymphocytic leukemia, lymphoma, less commonly with other disorders	Consult hematology

* Iron dextran: Dose (mL) = 0.0442 (desired Hb − observed Hb) × LBW (kg) + (0.26 × LBW). For LBW, see p 1. Administer test dose at 0.5 cc IM or IV solution (5 gtt/min). Wait 30–45 min. If tolerated, complete dose by slow IM injection ≤ 50 mg/min. By IV, dilute dose in 500 mL NS (45–60 cc/min).
** If level is borderline (200–300 pg/mL) and results would change treatment decision.

CANCER

Many older persons receive long-term drug therapy for cancers of the breast and prostate.

Breast Cancer

Prevention: Also see **Table 62**. Tamoxifen 20 mg po qd reduces breast cancer risk by 49% in women at high risk. For risk assessment see prevention section of http://www.cancer.gov/cancerinfo/prevention_genetics_causes/breast

Monitoring:
- History, physical
- LFTs, calcium every 4–6 mo for 5 yr, then yearly
- Annual mammography, pelvic, and FOBT

Pharmacotherapy: Postmenopausal women with estrogen receptor (ER) or progesterone receptor (PR) positive tumors at high risk for recurrence (tumors greater than 1 cm, or positive nodes) should be treated with oral adjuvant therapy for 5 yr, even when treated with chemotherapy. See **Table 36**.

Adjuvant Chemotherapy: Reduces recurrence risk for receptor-negative tumors. There is an additional 5% to 10% reduction in recurrence in ER- or PR-positive tumors treated with both tamoxifen and chemotherapy.

Therapy for Metastatic Bone Disease: Pamidronate or zoledronic acid reduces morbidity and delays time to onset of bone symptoms. Consult oncology.

Table 36. Oral Agents for Breast Cancer Treatment				
Class, Agent	Dosage	Formulations	Monitoring	Comment
Anti-estrogen Drugs				
Fulvestrant (*Faslodex*)	250 mg IM 1/mo in 1 or 2 injections	[Inj]	Blood chemistry, lipids	Has potent CYP3A4 inhibitors; GI reactions, anesthesia, pain (back, pelvic, headache), hot flushes
Tamoxifen* (*Nolvadex*)	20 mg po qd	[T: 10, 20]	Annual eye exam; endometrial cancer screening	Drug interactions: erythromycin, calcium channel blockers; ↑ risk of thrombosis
Toremifene (*Fareston*)	60 mg po qd	[T: 60]	CBC, Ca, LFTs, BUN, Cr	Drug interactions with CYP3A4–6 inhibitors and inducers (see **Table 6**); ↑ warfarin effect
Aromatase Inhibitors				
Letrozole† (*Femara*)	2.5 mg po qd	[T: 2.5]	Periodic CBC, LFTs, TSH	First-line therapy for hormone-responsive metastatic disease or tamoxifen failure

(*continues*)

Table 36. Oral Agents for Breast Cancer Treatment (cont.)				
Class, Agent	Dosage	Formulations	Monitoring	Comment
Anastrazole[†] (*Arimidex*)	1 mg po qd	[T: 1]	Periodic CBC, LFTs, lipids	First-line therapy for hormone-responsive metastatic disease or tamoxifen failure; may have more side effects

*Reduce dose if CrCl < 10 mL/min.

[†] In head-to-head trials, these aromatase inhibitors have lower recurrence rates than tamoxifen; both are more effective than tamoxifen in advanced inoperable disease. In one large randomized trial, aromatase inhibitors were superior to tamoxifen as adjuvant therapy in postmenopausal women.

Prostate Cancer
PSA: See **Table 62**.
Histology:
- Gleason score 2–6 has low 15–20 yr morbidity and mortality; watchful waiting usually appropriate.
- Gleason score $\geq$ 7, higher PSA and younger age associated with higher morbidity and mortality; best treatment strategy (surgery, radiation, androgen suppression, etc.) is not known.

Pharmacotherapy: Hormonal therapy is indicated in locally advanced $\geq$ stage III or T3 (tumor extension beyond the prostate capsule) and metastatic prostate cancer. Treatment of earlier stage disease is controversial. No luteinizing hormone-releasing hormone (LH–RH) agent is superior to others; they vary only in side-effect profile. Combining forms of androgen blockade has no advantage over monotherapy.

Table 37. Common Drugs for Prostate Cancer Therapy			
Class, Agent	Dosage	Metabolism	Side Effects
LH-RH agonists			
Goserelin acetate implant (*Zoladex*)	3.6 mg SC q 28 d or 10.8 mg q 3 mo	Rapid urinary and hepatic excretion, no dose adjustment in renal impairment	Side effects: hot flushes (60%), breast swelling, libido change, impotence, nausea
Leuprolide acetate (*Lupron Depot*)	7.5 mg IM q mo or 22.5 mg q 3 mo or 30 mg q 4 mo	Unknown; active metabolites for 4–12 wk, dose-dependent	Certain symptoms (obstruction, spinal cord compression, bone pain) may be exacerbated early in treatment; side effects: hot flushes (60%), edema (12%), pain (7%), nausea, vomiting, impotence, dyspnea, asthenia (all 5%), thrombosis, PE, MI (all 1%); headache as high as 32%

Table 37. Common Drugs for Prostate Cancer Therapy (cont.)			
Class, Agent	Dosage	Metabolism	Side Effects
Triptorelin (*Trelstar Depot, Trelstar LA*)	Depot: 375 mg q 28 d IM LA: 11.25 mg q 84 d IM	Hepatic metabolism and renal excretion (42% as intact peptide)	Hot flushes, ↑ glucose, ↓ Hgb, ↓ RBC, ↑ Alk Phos, ALT/AST, skeletal pain, ↑ BUN
Antiandrogens			
Bicalutamide (*Casodex*) [T: 50]	50 mg po qd	Metabolized in liver, excreted in urine; half-life 10 d at steady state	Class side effects: nausea, hot flushes, breast pain, gynecomastia, hematuria, diarrhea, liver enzyme elevations, galactorrhea; delayed light adaptation (nilutamide)
Flutamide (*Eulexin*) [C: 125]	125 mg cap 2 po q 8 h	Renally excreted; half-life 5–6 h	
Nilutamide (*Nilandron*) [T: 50]	300 mg for 30 d, then 150 mg po qd	80% protein bound; liver metabolism, renal excretion; half-life 40–60 h	

PNEUMONIA
Presentation
Can range from subtle signs such as lethargy, anorexia, dizziness, falls, and delirium to septic shock or adult respiratory distress syndrome. Pleuritic chest pain, dyspnea, productive cough, fever, chills, or rigors are not consistently present in older patients.

Evaluation and Assessment
- Physical examination: Respiratory rate > 20 breaths/min; low BP, chest sounds may be minimal, absent, or consistent with CHF; temperature: 20% will be afebrile.
- CXR: Infiltrate may not be present on initial film if the patient is dehydrated.
- Sputum Gram's stain and culture (optional per ATS guidelines)
- CBC with differential: Up to 50% of patients have a normal white blood cell count, but 95% have a left shift.
- BUN, creatinine, electrolytes, glucose
- Blood culture × 2
- Oxygenation: arterial blood gas or oximetry
- Test for *Mycobacterium tuberculosis* with acid fast bacilli strain and culture in selected patients.
- Test for *Legionella* spp in patients who are seriously ill without an alternative diagnosis, immunocompromised, nonresponsive to β-lactam antibiotics, have clinical features suggesting this diagnosis, or in outbreak setting. Urinary antigen testing is highly specific for serotype 1 but lacks specificity for other serotypes. Value and use vary by geographic region.
- Thoracentesis (if moderate to large effusion)

Aggravating Factors
- Age-related changes in pulmonary reserve
- Alcoholism
- Altered mental status
- Comorbid conditions that alter gag reflexes or ciliary transport
- COPD or other lung disease
- Heart disease
- Malnutrition
- Medications: Immunosuppressants, sedatives, anticholinergic or other agents that dry secretions, agents that decrease gastric pH
- Nasogastric tubes

Expected Organisms (in order of frequency of occurrence)

Community-Acquired:
Streptococcus pneumoniae
Respiratory viruses
Haemophilus influenzae
Gram-negative bacteria
Chlamydia pneumoniae
Moraxella catarrhalis
Legionella spp
M tuberculosis
Endemic fungi

Nursing-Home–Acquired:
S pneumoniae
Gram-negative bacteria
Staphylococcus aureus
Anaerobes
H influenzae
Group B streptococcus
Chlamydia pneumoniae

Hospital-Acquired:
Gram-negative bacteria
Anaerobes
Gram-positive bacteria
Fungi

Supportive Management
- Chest percussion
- Inhaled β-adrenergic agonists
- Mechanical ventilation (if indicated)
- Oxygen as indicated
- Rehydration

Empiric Antibiotic Therapy (see **Table 45**)

Community-Acquired (oral route):
(2nd gen ceph or β-lact or FLQ*) ± macro if Legionella spp suspected

Community-Acquired with Hospitalization (oral or IV):
(2nd, 3rd, or 4th gen ceph or β-lact or FLQ*) ± erythromycin or other macro if Legionella spp suspected

Severe Community-Acquired with Hospitalization (IV):
Macro + ceftazidime or cefepime or other antipseudomonal agent

Nursing-Home Acquired (IV):
[(1st or 2nd gen ceph or ureidopenicillin) + AG] ± pen G, clinda, or vanco
or 3rd or 4th gen ceph ± AG ± pen G, clinda, or vanco
or ureidopenicillin + AG
or vanco + clinda + AG
For the oral route: see Community-Acquired (above) ± FLQ

Hospital-Acquired (IV):
[3rd or 4th gen ceph + clinda or pen G] ± AG
or ureidopenicillin + AG or other antipseudomonal agent
or 1st or 2nd gen ceph + AG
or vanco + clinda + AG
or ureidopenicillin + 2nd gen ceph
or β-lact + antipseudomonal agent
For hospital- or nursing-home-acquired pneumonia, a macro, tetracycline, or FLQ may be added or substituted when Legionella spp or Mycobacterium pneumonia is suspected.

* Refers to FLQ with enhanced activity against *S. pneumonia* (levofloxacin, sparfloxacin, moxifloxacin).
Note: AG = aminoglycoside; β-lact = β-lactam/ β-lactamase inhibitor; ceph = cephalosporin; clinda = clindamycin; FLQ = fluoroquinolone; gen = generation; macro = macrolide; pen G = penicillin G; vanco = vancomycin.

Note: The empiric use of vancomycin should be reserved for patients with a serious allergy to β-lactam antibiotics or for patients from environments in which methicillin-resistant *S aureus* is known to be a problem pathogen. For all cases, antimicrobial therapy should be individualized once Gram's stain or culture results are known.

URINARY TRACT INFECTION OR UROSEPSIS

Definition
Bacteriuria: Presence of significant number of bacteria without reference to symptoms
UTI: Symptomatic bacteriuria

Table 38. Quantitative Urine Microbiology for Diagnosis of Urinary Tract Infection	
Clinical Presentation	**Quantitative Microbiology**
Asymptomatic	Same organism(s) $\geq 10^5$ cfu/mL on 2 consecutive cultures
Pyelonephritis or fever with localized symptoms	$\geq 10^4$ cfu/mL
Acute lower tract symptoms	$\geq 10^3$ cfu/mL of uropathogen
Specimen collected from:	
External collecting device (men only)	$\geq 10^5$ cfu/mL
Aspirated indwelling catheter	$\geq 10^3$ cfu/mL

Source: Nicolle LE. Urinary tract infections in the elderly. In: Hazzard WR, Blass JP, Ettinger WH, et al., eds., *Principles of Geriatric Medicine and Gerontology*, 3rd ed. New York: McGraw-Hill Publishing; 1994. Reprinted with permission of The McGraw-Hill Companies.

Risk Factors
- Abnormalities in function or anatomy of the urinary tract
- Catheterization or recent instrumentation
- Comorbid conditions (eg, diabetes mellitus, BPH)
- Female gender
- Limited functional status

Assessment and Evaluation
Choice is based on presenting symptoms and severity of illness.
- Urinalysis with culture (do not obtain specimen from catheter bag)
- Blood culture × 2
- BUN, creatinine, electrolytes
- CBC with differential

Expected Organisms
Noncatheterized Patients: Most common: *Escherichia coli, Proteus* spp, *Klebsiella* spp, *Providencia* spp, *Citrobacter* spp, *Enterobacter* spp, and *Pseudomonas aeruginosa* if recent antibiotic exposure, known colonization, or known institutional flora
Nursing-Home–Catheterized Patients: *Enterobacter* spp and gram-negative bacteria

Empiric Antibiotic Management
Duration should be at least 7–10 d.
Community-Acquired or Nursing-Home–Acquired Cystitis or Uncomplicated UTI (Oral Route): TMP/SMZ DS, cephalexin, ampicillin, or amoxicillin. Amoxicillin/clavulanic acid should be reserved for patients with sulfa allergy and in settings where β-lactam resistance is known. Fluoroquinolones should be reserved for patients with allergies to sulpha, β-lactams, or in settings where resistance is known.
Suspected Urosepsis (IV Route): Third-generation cephalosporin plus aminoglycoside, aztreonam, or fluoroquinolone ± aminoglycoside.

Vancomycin should be used in patients with severe β-lactam allergy.

HERPES ZOSTER ("SHINGLES")
Definition
Cutaneous vesicular eruptions followed by radicular pain secondary to the recrudescence of varicella zoster virus.

Clinical Manifestations
- An abrupt onset of pain along a specific dermatome (see **Figure 1**)
- Macular, erythematous rash after ~3 d which becomes vesicular and pustular (Tzanck cell test positive), crusts over and clears in 10–14 d
- Complications: post-herpetic neuralgia, visual loss or blindness if ophthalmic involvement

Pharmacologic Management
When started within 72 h of the rash's appearance, antiviral therapy decreases the severity and duration of the acute illness and possibly shortens the duration and reduces the risk of post-herpetic neuralgias. Corticosteroids may also decrease the risk and severity of post-herpetic neuralgias. (See p 111 for treatment of post-herpetic neuralgia.)

Table 39. Antiviral Treatments for Herpes Zoster			
Agent, Route	**Dosage**	**Formulations**	**Comment**
Acyclovir (*Zovirax*)			
Oral	800 mg 5 ×/d for 7–10 d	[T: 400, 800; C: 200; S: 200 mg/5 mL]	Reduce dose when CrCl* < 50 mL/min
IV**	10 mg/kg q 8 h for 7–10 d	[500 mg/10 mL]	
Famciclovir (*Famvir*)			
Oral	500 mg q 8 h for 7–10 d	[T: 125, 250, 500]	Reduce dose when CrCl* < 60 mL/min
Valacyclovir† (*Valtrex*)			
Oral	1000 mg q 8 h for 7–10 d	[C: 500, 1000]	Reduce dose when CrCl* < 50 mL/min

* The CrCl listed is the threshold below which the dose or frequency should be reduced. See alternative reference or the drug's package insert for detailed dosing guidelines.
** Use IV for serious illness, ophthalmic infection, or patients who cannot take oral medication.
† Preferred to po acyclovir; pro-drug of acyclovir with serum concentrations equal to IV.

INFLUENZA
Vaccine Prevention (ACIP Guidelines)
Yearly vaccination is recommended for all persons ≥ 65 years and all residents and staff of nursing homes, or residential or long-term-care facilities. Nursing-home residents admitted during the winter months after the completion of the vaccination program should be vaccinated at admission if they have not already been vaccinated. The influenza vaccine is contraindicated in persons with an anaphylactic hypersensitivity to eggs or any other component of the vaccine. Dose: 0.5 mL IM × 1 in the fall (Oct–Nov) for residents in the northern hemisphere.

Pharmacologic Prophylaxis and Treatment with Antiviral Agents
Indications:
- Prevention (during an influenza outbreak): persons who are not vaccinated, are immunodeficient, or may spread the virus
- Prophylaxis: during 2 wk required to develop antibodies for persons vaccinated after an outbreak of influenza A
- Reduction of symptoms, duration of illness when started within the first 48 h of symptoms
- During epidemic outbreaks in nursing homes

Duration: Treatment of symptoms: 3–5 d or for 24–48 h after symptoms resolve. Prophylaxis during outbreak: Minimum 2 wk or until ~1 wk after end of outbreak.

Table 40. Antiviral Treatment of Influenza	
Agent	**Dosage**
Amantadine (*Symmetrel*)	100 mg po daily*
Oseltamivir (*Tamiflu*)**	Treatment: 75 mg po bid × 5 d (75 mg po qd if CrCl 10–30 mL/min) Prophylaxis: 75 mg po qd × ≥ 7 d up to 2 wk (75 mg po qod if CrCl 10–30 mL/min)
Rimantadine (*Flumadine*)	100 mg po qd for frail elderly and nursing-home residents 200 mg po qd for other adults, including those ≥ 65 yr Decrease dose to 100 mg if side effects appear
Zanamivir (*Relenza*)**†	2 × 5-mg inhalations q 12 h × 5 d Give doses on 1st d at least 2 h apart

* Dose adjustments for renal function, CrCl (mL/min): ≥ 30 = 100 mg daily; 20–29 = 200 mg 2 ×/wk; 10–19 = 100 mg 3 × /wk; < 10 = 200 mg alternating with 100 mg q 7 d.
** Must be started within 2 d of symptom onset.
† Do not use in patients with COPD or asthma.

INFECTIOUS TUBERCULOSIS
Tuberculosis (TB) in elderly patients may be the reactivation of old disease or a new infection due to exposure to an infected individual. Treatment recommendations differ; if a new infection is suspected or the patient has risk factors for resistant organisms, then bacterial sensitivities must be determined.

Risk or Reactivating Factors
- Chronic institutionalization
- Corticosteroid use
- Diabetes mellitus
- Malignancy
- Malnutrition
- Renal failure

Risk Factors for Resistant Organisms
- HIV infection
- Homelessness, institutionalization (other than a nursing home)
- IV drug abuse
- Origin from geographic regions with a high prevalence of resistance (New York, Mexico, Southeast Asia)
- Exposure to INH-resistant TB or history of failed chemotherapy
- Previous treatment for TB
- AFB-positive sputum smears after 2 mo of treatment
- Positive cultures after 4 mo of treatment

Diagnosis
- PPD with booster 5-TU subdermal; read in 48–72 h; repeat in 1–2 wk if negative (see **Table 41**)
- CXR

Treatment
Latent Infection:

Table 41. Identification of Patients at High Risk of Developing TB Who Would Benefit From Treatment of Latent Infection	
Population	**Minimum Induration Considered a Positive Test**
Low risk: testing generally not indicated	15 mm
Residents and employees of hospitals, nursing homes, and long-term facilities for elderly persons, residential facilities for AIDS patients, and homeless shelters	
Recent immigrants (< 5 yr) from high-prevalence countries	10 mm
Injection drug users	
Persons with silicosis, diabetes mellitus, chronic renal failure, leukemia, lymphoma, carcinoma of the head, neck, or lung, weight loss of ≥ 10%, gastrectomy or jejunoileal bypass	
Recent contact with TB patients	
Fibrotic changes on CXR consistent with prior TB	
Immunosuppressed (receiving the equivalent of ≥ 15 mg/d of prednisone for ≥ 1 mo) or organ transplants	5 mm
HIV-positive patients	

Table 42. Treatment of Latent Tuberculosis	
Drug	**Dose and Duration**
INH*	5 mg/kg/d (maximum 300 mg/d) for 6 or 9 mo; or 15 mg/kg/d (maximum 900 mg/d) 2 × /wk with directly observed therapy (DOT) for 6 or 9 mo
RIF plus PZA†	10 mg/kg/d (maximum 600 mg/d) 15–20 mg/kg/d (maximum 2 gm/d) daily for 2 mo
or RIF plus PZA†	10 mg/kg/d (maximum 600 mg/d) 2 × /wk with DOT for 2–3 mo 50 mg/kg/d (maximum 4 gm/d) 2 × /wk with DOT for 2–3 mo
RIF	10 mg/kg/d (maximum 600 mg/d) for 4 mo

Note: INH = isoniazid; PZA = pyrozinamide; RIF = rifampin.

* The preferred treatment for patients not infected with HIV.

† Use the combination therapy with caution, as the 2-mo regimen has been associated with liver injury. Obtain a serum aminotransferase, and bilirubin at baseline and 2, 4, and 6 wk of treatment. For additional information, see *MMWR* 2001; 50(34):733–735 or http://www.ajrccm.atsjournals.org/cgi/content/full/161/4/S1/S221/DC1

Source: Data from: American Thoracic Society. Targeted tuberculin testing and treatment of latent tuberculosis. *Am J Respir Crit Care Med* 2000;161:S221–S247 (also available at http://www.atsjournal.org).

Active Infection:

Initial treatment options for adults with active *Mycobacterium tuberculosis* (note: INH = isoniazid; PZA = pyrazinamide; RIF = rifampin):

- Daily INH, RIF, and PZA X 8 wk, followed by 16 wk of INH and RIF daily or 2–3 times/wk. Add ethambutol or streptomycin to the initial regimen if area INH resistance rate is not documented to be < 4%; continue until susceptibility to INH and RIF are known.
- Daily INH, RIF, PZA, and ethambutol or streptomycin X 2 wk followed by all agents given 2 times/wk by daily observed therapy X 6 wk followed by INH and RIF 2 times/wk X 16 wk by daily observed therapy.
- INH, RIF, PZA, and ethambutol or streptomycin 3 times/wk for 6 mo by daily observed therapy.

Table 43. Dosing for Treatment Options for Active Tuberculosis				
Agent	Route	Daily	2/Wk	3/Wk
INH	po, IM	300 mg*	15 mg/kg*	15 mg/kg*
RIF	po, IM	600 mg**	600 mg**	600 mg**
PZA	po	1.5 g (< 50 kg) 2 g (51–74 kg) 2.5 g (≥ 75 kg)	2.0 g (< 50 kg) 2.5 g (51–74 kg) 3.0 g (≥ 75 kg)	2.0 g (< 50 kg) 2.5 g (51–74 kg) 3.0 g (≥ 75 kg)
Ethambutol	po	15–25 mg/kg†	50 mg/kg	30 mg/kg
Streptomycin		10 mg/kg	—	—

* Maximums: daily = 300 mg; 2/wk = 900 mg; 3/wk = 900 mg.
** Maximums: daily = 600 mg; 2/wk = 600 mg; 3/wk= 600 mg.
† Maximum: daily = 2.5 g.

ANTIBIOTIC-ASSOCIATED DIARRHEA
(Antibiotic-associated pseudomembranous colitis, or AAPMC)

Definition
A specific form of *Clostridium difficile* pseudomembranous colitis

Risk Factors
Almost any oral or parenteral antibiotic and several antineoplastic agents, including cyclophosphamide, doxorubicin, fluorouracil, methotrexate.

Presentation
- Abdominal pain, cramping
- Dehydration
- Diarrhea (can be bloody)
- Fecal leukocytes
- Fever (100–105°F)
- Hypoalbuminemia
- Hypovolemia
- Leukocytosis

Symptoms appear a few days after starting to 10 wk after discontinuing the offending agent.

Diagnosis

- Isolation of *C difficile* or its toxin from symptomatic patient. Three negative stools are needed to exclude diagnosis.
- Lower endoscopy; however, lesions may be scattered.

Treatment

- Discontinue offending agent if possible.
- Metronidazole (*Flagyl*) 250 mg po qid or 500 mg po tid × 10 d or vancomycin 125–500 mg po qid × 10 d.
- Treat diarrhea with cholestyramine resin (eg, *Questran*) 4 g 1–6 ×/d to adsorb toxin.
- Avoid opiates or other agents that will slow GI motility.

Recurrence

Relapse seen in 10% to 20% of patients 1–4 wk after treatment (spore-producing organism). Re-treat with same regimen or use alternative.

Table 44. Monitoring Aminoglycosides and Vancomycin

Antimicrobial	Therapeutic Concentration	
	Peak (μg/mL)	Trough (μg/mL)
Amikacin	25–30	4–8 (< 5*)
Gentamicin or tobramycin	4–8	<2 (< 0.5*)
Vancomycin	20–40	5–10

Note: Draw peak concentrations 30 min after completion of a 30-min infusion or at 1 h following initiation of infusion or IM injection. Draw trough within 30 min of next dose.
* For once-daily or extended-interval dosing.

Table 45. Antibiotics

Class, *Subclass*, Antimicrobial	Route of Elimination (%)	Dosage	Adjust When CrCl* Is: (mL/min)	Formulations
β–**Lactams**				
Penicillins				
Amoxicillin (*Amoxil*)	K (80)	po: 250 mg–1 g q 8 h	< 50	[T: film coated 500, 875] [C: 250, 500] [ChT: 125, 200, 250, 400] [S: 125, 200, 250, 400 mg/5 mL]
Ampicillin	K (90)	po: 250–500 mg q 6 h IM/IV: 1–2 g q 4–6 h	< 30	[C: 250, 500] [S: 125, 250 mg/5 mL] [Inj]
Penicillin G	K L (30)	IV: 3–5 × 10⁶ U q 4–6 h IM: 0.6–2.4 × 10⁶ U q 6–12 h	< 30	[Inj] [procaine for IM]
Penicillin VK	K, L	po: 125–500 mg q 6 h		[T: 125, 250, 500] [S: 125, 250 mg/5 mL]

(continues)

Table 45. Antibiotics (cont.)				
Class, *Subclass*, Antimicrobial ⟳	Route of Elimination (%)	Dosage	Adjust When CrCl* Is: (mL/min)	Formulations
Carbenicillin indanyl sodium (*Geocillin*)	K (80–99)	po: 382–764 mg q 6 h	< 50	[T: 382]
Ureidopenicillins				
Penicillinase-resistant nafcillin	L	IM: 500 mg q 4–6 h IV: 500 mg–2 g q q 4–6 h	NA	[Inj]
Oxacillin (*Bactocill*)	K	po: 500 mg–1 g q 4–6 h IM, IV: 250 mg–2 g q 6–12 h	< 10	[C: 250, 500] [S: 250 mg/5 mL] [Inj]
Aztreonam (*Azactam*)	K (70)	IM: 500 mg–1 g q 8–12 h IV: 500 mg–2 g q 6–12 h	< 30	[Inj]
Meropenem (*Merrem IV*)	K (75), L (25)	IV: 1 g q 8 h	≤ 50	[Inj]
Imipenem-Cilastatin (*Primaxin*)	K (70)	IM: 500 mg–1 g q 8–12 h IV: 500 mg–2 g q 6–12 h	< 70	[Inj]
Amoxicillin–Clavulanate (*Augmentin*)	K	po: 250 mg q 8 h, 500 mg q 12 h, 875 mg q 12 h	< 30	[T: 250, 500, 875] [ChT: 125, 200, 250, 400] [S: 125, 200, 250, 400 mg/5 mL]
Ampicillin–Sulbactam (*Unasyn*)	K (85)	IM, IV: 1–2 g q q 6–8 h	< 30	[Inj]
Piperacillin–Tazobactam (*Zosyn*)	K	IV: 3.375 g q 6 h	< 40	[Inj]
Ticarcillin–Clavulanate (*Timentin*)	K, L	IV: 3 g q 4–6 h	< 60	[Inj]
First-Generation Cephalosporins				
Cefadroxil (*Duricef*)	K (90)	po: 500 mg–1 g q 12 h	< 50	[C: 500; T: 1 g] [S: 125, 250, 500 mg/5 mL]
Cefazolin (*Ancef, Kefzol*)	K (80–100)	IM, IV: 500 mg–2 g q q 8 h	< 55	[Inj]
Cephalexin (*Keflex*)	K (80–100)	po: 250 mg–1 g q 6 h	< 40	[C: 250, 500] [T: 250, 500; 1 g] [S: 125, 250 mg/5 mL]
Cephalothin (*Keflin*)	K (50–75)	IM, IV: 500 mg–2 g q q 4–6 h	< 50	[Inj]
Cephapirin (*Cefadyl*)	K (60–85)	IM, IV: 1–3 g q 6 h	< 10	[Inj]
Cephradine (*Anspor*)	K (80–90)	po, IM, IV: 500 mg–2 g q q 6 h	< 20	[C: 250, 500] [T: 1 g] [S: 125, 250 mg/5 mL] [Inj]
Second-Generation Cephalosporins				
Cefaclor (*Ceclor*)	K (80)	po: 250–500 mg q 8 h	< 50	[C: 250, 500] [S: 125, 187, 250, 375 mg/5 mL] [T: ER 375, 500]

Table 45. Antibiotics (cont.)				
Class, *Subclass,* Antimicrobial	Route of Elimination (%)	Dosage	Adjust When CrCl* Is: (mL/min)	Formulations
Cefamandole (*Mandol*)	K	IM, IV: 1–3 g q 6 h	< 80	[Inj]
Cefmetazole (*Zefazone*)	K (85)	IV: 2 g q 6–12 h	< 90	[Inj]
Cefotetan (*Cefotan*)	K (80)	IM, IV: 1–3 g q 12 h or 1–2 g q 24 h (UTI)	< 30	[Inj]
Cefoxitin (*Mefoxin*)	K (85)	IM, IV: 1–2 g q 6–8 h	< 50	[Inj]
Cefprozil (*Cefzil*)	K (60–70)	po: 250–500 mg q 12–24 h	< 30	[T: 250, 500] [S: 125, 250 mg/5 mL]
Cefuroxime axetil (*Ceftin*)	K (66–100)	po: 125–500 mg q 12 h IM, IV: 750 mg–1.5 g q 6 h	< 30	[T: 125, 250, 500] [S: 125, 150 mg/5 mL] [Inj]
Loracarbef (*Lorabid*)	K	po: 200–400 mg q 12–24 h	< 50	[C: 200, 400] [S: 100, 200 mg/5 mL]
Third-Generation Cephalosporins				
Cefdinir (*Omnicef*)	K	po: 300 mg bid or 600 qd × 10 d	< 30	[C: 300]
Cefixime (*Suprax*)	K (50)	po: 400 mg q 24 h	< 60	[T: 200, 400] [S: 125 mg/5 ml.] [S: 100 mg/5 mL]
Cefoperazone (*Cefobid*)	L, K (25)	IM, IV: 1–2 g q 12 h	Adjust in cirrhosis	[Inj]
Cefotaxime (*Claforan*)	K, L	IM, IV: 1–2 g q 6–12 h	< 20	[Inj]
Cefpodoxime (*Vantin*)	K (80)	po: 100–400 mg q 12 h	< 30	[T: 100, 250] [S: 50, 100 mg/5 mL]
Ceftazidime (*Ceptaz, Fortaz*)	K	IM, IV: 500 mg–2 g q 8–12 h UTI: 250–500 mg q 12 h	< 50	[Inj]
Ceftibuten (*Cedax*)	K (65–70)	po: 400 mg q 24 h	< 50	[C: 400] [S: 100, 200 mg/5 mL]
Ceftizoxime (*Cefizox*)	K (100)	IM, IV: 500 mg–2 g q 4–12 h	< 80	[Inj]
Ceftriaxone (*Rocephin*)	K (33–65)	IM, IV: 1–2 g q 12–24 h	NA	[Inj]
Fourth-Generation Cephalosporins				
Cefepime (*Maxipime*)	K (85)	IV: 500 mg–2 g q 12 h	< 60	[Inj]
Aminoglycosides (see **Table 44** for monitoring levels)				
Amikacin (*Amikin*)	K (95)	IM, IV: 15–20 mg/kg/d divided q 12–24 h; 15–20 mg/kg q 24–48 h		[Inj]
Gentamicin (*Garamycin*)	K (95)	IM, IV: 2–5 mg/kg/d divided q 12–24 h; 5–7 mg/kg q 24–48 h		[Inj] [ophth sus, oint]
Streptomycin	K (90)	IM, IV: 10 mg/kg/d not to exceed 750 mg/d	< 50	[Inj]
Tobramycin (*Nebcin*)	K (95)	IM, IV: 2–5 mg/kg/d divided q 12–24 h; 5–7 mg/kg q 24–48 h		[Inj] [ophth sus, oint]

(*continues*)

Table 45. Antibiotics (cont.)

Class, *Subclass*, Antimicrobial	Route of Elimination (%)	Dosage	Adjust When CrCl* Is: (mL/min)	Formulations
Macrolides				
Azithromycin (*Zithromax*)	L	po: 500 mg day 1, then 250 mg IV: 500 mg qd	NA	[C: 250] [S: 100, 200 mg/5 mL, 1 g (single-dose pk)] [T: 600]
Clarithromycin (*Biaxin, Biaxin XL*)	L, K (20–30)	po: 250–500 mg q 12 h ER: 1000 mg q 24 h	< 30	[S: 125, 250 mg/5 mL] [T: 250, 500] [ER: 500]
Dirithromycin (*Dynabac*)	L, F	po: 500 mg qd with food	NA	[T: 250]
Erythromycin	L	po: Base 333 mg q 8 h Estolate, stearate or base: 250–500 mg q 6–12 h Ethylsuccinate: 400–800 mg q 6–12 h IV: 15–20 mg/kg/d divided q 6 h	NA	[Base: C, T: 250, 333, 500] [Estolate: 250] [S: 125, 250 mg/5 mL] [T: 500] Ethylsuccinate: [S: 100, 200, 400 mg/5 mL] [T: 400] [ChT: 200] [Stearate: T: 250, 500] [Inj]
Quinolones				
Cinoxacin (*Cinobac*)	K (60)	po: 500 bid	< 80	[C: 250, 500]
Ciprofloxacin (*Cipro*)	K (30–50), L, F (20–40)	po: 250–750 mg q 12 h IV: 200–400 mg q 12 h ophth: see **Table 77 note**	po: < 50 IV: < 30	[T: 100, 250, 500, 750] [S: 250 mg/5 mL, 500 mg/5 mL] [ophth sol: 3.5 mg/5 mL] [Inj]
Enoxacin (*Penetrex*)	K, L (15–20)	po: 200 mg q 12 h × 7d or 400 mg q 12 h × 14 d	≤ 30	[T: 200, 400]
Gatifloxacin (*Tequin*)	K (95), F (5)	po, IV: 200–400 mg qd × 7–10 d	< 40	[T: 200, 400] [Inj]
Levofloxacin (*Levaquin*)	K	po, IV: 250–500 mg q 24 h	< 50	[T: 250, 500]
Lomefloxacin (*Maxaquin*)	K	po: 400 mg q 24 h	< 40	[T: 400]
Moxifloxacin (*Avelox*)	L (~55), F (25), K (20)	po: 400 mg q 24 h	NA	[T: 400]
Norfloxacin (*Noraxin*)	K (30), F (30)	po: 400 mg q 12 h ophth: see **Table 77 note**	< 30	[T: 400] [ophth: 0.3%]
Ofloxacin (*Roxin*)	K	po, IV: 200–400 mg q 12–24 h ophth: see **Table 77 note**	< 50	[T: 200, 300, 400] [ophth: 0.3%] [Inj]
Sparfloxacin (*Zagam*)	L	po: 400 mg day 1, then 200 mg q 24 h	< 50	[T: 200]
Trovafloxacin (*Trovan*)	L	po, IV: 200 mg q 24 h × 10–14 d	NA	[T: 100, 200] [Inj]

Table 45. Antibiotics (cont.)				
Class, *Subclass*, Antimicrobial	Route of Elimination (%)	Dosage	Adjust When CrCl* Is: (mL/min)	Formulations
Tetracyclines				
Doxycycline (eg, *Vibramycin*)	K (25), F (30)	po, IV: 100–200 mg/d given q 12–24 h	NA	[C: 50, 100] [T: 50, 100] [S:25 mg/5 mL, 50 mg/5 mL] [Inj]
Minocycline (*Minocin*)	K	po, IV: 200 mg × 1, 100 mg q 12 h	NA	[C: 50, 100] [S: 50 mg/5 mL] [Inj]
Tetracycline	K (60)	po, IV: 250–500 mg q 6–12 h	NA	[C: 100, 250, 500] [T: 250, 500] [S: 125 mg/5 mL] [ophth: oint, sus] [topical: oint, sol]
Other Antibiotics				
Chloramphenicol (*Chloromycetin*)	L (90)	po, IV: 50 mg/kg/d given q 6 h; maximum: 4 g/d		[C: 250] [topical] [ophth] [Inj]
Clindamycin (*Cleocin*)	L (90)	po: 150–450 mg q 6–8 h; maximum: 1.8 g/d IM, IV: 1.2–1.8 g/d given q 8–12 h; maximum: 3.6 g/d	NA	[C: 75, 150, 300] [S: 75 mg/5 mL] [cre, vaginal: 2%] [gel, topical: 1%] [Inj]
Co-trimoxazole (TMP/SMZ, *Bactrim*)	K, L	Doses based on the trimethoprim component: po: 1 double-strength tablet q 12 h. IV: sepsis: 20 TMP/kg/d given q 6 h	≤ 50	[T: SMZ 400; TMP 80] [double-strength: SMZ 800; TMP 160] [S: SMZ 200; TMP 40 mg/5 mL] [Inj]
Linezolid (*Zyvox*)	L (65), K (30)	po: 400–600 mg q 12 h IV: 600 mg q 12 h	NA	[T: 400, 600] [S: 100 mg/5 mL] [Inj]
Metronidazole (*Flagyl, MetraGel*)	L (30–60), K (20–40), F (6–15)	po: 250–750 mg q 6–8 h Vaginal: 1 applicator full (375 mg) qhs or bid Topical: Apply bid	≤ 10	[T: 250, 500] [ER: 750] [C: 375] [gel, topical: 0.75% (30g)] [gel, vaginal: 0.75% (70g)] [Inj]
Nitrofurantoin (*Macrodantin*)	L (60), K (40)	po: 50–100 mg q 6 h	Do not use if < 40	[C: 25, 50, 100] [S: 25 mg/5 mL]
Quinupristin/ dalfopristin (*Synercid*)	L, B, F (75), K (15–19)	Vancomycin-resistant *E faecium*: IV: 7.5 mg/ kg q 8 h Complicated skin or skin structure infection: 7.5 mg/kg q 12 h	NA	[Inj]

(continues)

Table 45. Antibiotics (cont.)				
Class, *Subclass*, Antimicrobial	Route of Elimination (%)	Dosage	Adjust When CrCl* Is: (mL/min)	Formulations
Vancomycin (*Vancocin*) (see **Table 44** for monitoring levels)	K (80–90)	po: *C difficile:* 125–500 mg q 6–8 h IV: 500 mg–1 g q q 8–24 h		[C: 125, 250] [Inj]
Antifungals				
Amphotericin B (*Fungizone*)	K	IV: test dose: 1 mg infused over 20–30 min; if tolerated, initial therapeutic dose is 0.25 mg/kg; the daily dose can be increased by 0.25-mg/kg increments on each subsequent day until the desired daily dose is reached Maintenance dose: IV: 0.25–1 mg/kg/d or 1.5 mg/kg qod; do not exceed 1.5 mg/kg/d	**	[topical: cre, lot, oint 3%] [Inj]
Caspofungin (*Cancidas*)	L	Initial: 70 mg infused over 1 h, then 50 mg/d over 1 hr	—	[Inj]
Fluconazole (*Diflucan*)	K (80)	po, IV: first dose 200– 400 mg, then 100– 400 mg qd for 14 d–12 wk, depending on indication. Vaginal candidiasis: 150 mg as a single dose	< 50	[T: 50, 100, 150, 200] [S: 10 and 40 mg/mL] [Inj]
Flucytosine (*Ancobon*)	K (75–90)	po: 50–150 mg/kg/d divided q 6 h	< 50	[C: 250, 500]
Griseofulvin (*Fulvicin P/G, Grifulvin V*)	L	po: Microsize: 500– 1000 mg/d in single or divided doses Ultramicrosize: 330– 375 mg/d in single or divided doses Duration based on indication	NA	Microsize: [C: 125, 250] [S: 125 mg/5 mL] [T: 250, 500] Ultramicrosize: [T: 125, 165, 250, 330]
Itraconazole (*Sporanox*)	L	po: 200–400 mg/d; doses > 200 mg/d should be divided. Life-threatening infections: loading dose: 200 mg tid (600 mg/d) should be given for the first 3 d of therapy IV: 200 mg bid × 4 d, then 200 mg qd	< 30	[C: 100] [S: 100 mg/10 mL] [Inj]

Table 45. Antibiotics (cont.)				
Class, *Subclass,* Antimicrobial	Route of Elimination (%)	Dosage	Adjust When CrCl* Is: (mL/min)	Formulations
Ketoconazole (*Nizoral*)	L, F	po: 200–400 mg qd shp: 2/wk × 4 wk with at least 3 d between each shp Topical: apply qd–bid	NA	[cre: 2%] [shp: 2%] [T: 200]
Miconazole (*Monistat IV*)	L, F	IT: 20 mg q 1–2 d IV: initial: 200 mg, then 1.2–3.6 g/d divided q 8 h for up to 2 wk	NA	[Inj]

Note: NA = not applicable.
* The CrCl listed is the threshold below which the dose or frequency should be adjusted. See alternative reference or the drug package insert for detailed dosing guidelines.
** Adjust dose if decreased renal function is due to the drug, or give every other day.

MALNUTRITION

DEFINITION
There is no uniformly accepted definition of malnutrition in older persons. Some commonly used definitions include the following:

Community-Dwelling Men and Women
- Involuntary weight loss (eg, $\geq$ 10 lb over 6 months, $\geq$ 4% over 1 yr)
- Abnormal body mass index (eg, BMI > 27; BMI < 22)
- Hypoalbuminemia (eg, $\leq$ 3.8 g/dL)
- Hypocholesterolemia (eg, < 160 mg/dL)
- Specific vitamin or micronutrient deficiencies (eg, vitamin B_{12})

Hospitalized Patients
- Dietary intake (eg, < 50% of estimated needed caloric intake)
- Hypoalbuminemia (eg, < 3.5 g/dL)
- Hypocholesterolemia (eg, < 160 mg/dL)

Nursing-Home Patients (Triggered by the Minimum Data Set)
- Weight loss of $\geq$ 5% in past 30 d; $\geq$ 10% in 180 d
- Dietary intake of < 75% at most meals

EVALUATION
Multidimensional Assessment
In the absence of valid nutrition screening instruments, clinicians should focus on whether the following issues may be affecting nutritional status:
- Economic barriers to securing food
- Availability of sufficiently high-quality food
- Dental problems that prohibit ingesting high-quality food
- Medical illnesses that
  - interfere with digestion or absorption of food
  - increase nutritional requirements
  - require dietary restrictions (eg, low-sodium diet or npo)
- Functional disability that interferes with shopping, preparing meals, or feeding
- Food preferences or cultural beliefs that interfere with adequate food intake
- Poor appetite
- Depressive symptoms

Anthropometrics
Weight on each visit and yearly height (see p 1)

Biochemical Markers
Serum Proteins: All may drop precipitously because of trauma, sepsis, or major infection.
- Albumin (half-life 18–20 d) has prognostic value in all settings.
- Transferrin (half-life 7 d)
- Prealbumin (half-life 48 h) may be valuable in monitoring nutritional recovery.

Serum Cholesterol (Low or Falling Levels): Has prognostic value in all settings but may not be nutritionally mediated.

MANAGEMENT
Calculating Basic Energy (Caloric) and Fluid Requirements
- WHO energy estimates for adults aged 60 yr and older:
  - Women (10.5) (weight in kg) + 596
  - Men (13.5) (weight in kg) + 487
- Harris-Benedict energy requirement equations:
  - Women 655 + (9.6) (weight in kg) + (1.7) (height in cm) − (4.7) (age in yr)
  - Men 66 + (13.7) (weight in kg) + (5.0) (height in cm) − (6.8) (age in yr)

Depending on activity and physiologic stress levels, these basic requirements may need to be increased (eg, 25% for sedentary or mild, 50% for moderate, and 100% for intense or severe activity or stress).
- Fluid requirements for older persons without cardiac or renal disease are approximately 30 mL/kg of body weight/d.

Appetite Stimulants
- No drugs are FDA approved for weight loss in older persons.
- Dronabinol and megestrol acetate have been effective in promoting weight gain in younger adults with specific conditions (eg, AIDS, cancer).
- A minority of patients receiving mirtazapine report appetite stimulation and weight gain.
- All drugs used for appetite have substantial potential side effects.

Oral and Enteral Formulas
Many formulas are available (see **Table 46**). Read the content labels and choose on the basis of calories/mL, protein, fiber, lactose, and fluid load.
- Oral: Many (eg, *Carnation Instant Breakfast, Health Shake*) are milk-based and provide approximately 1.0–1.5 calories/mL.
- Enteral: Commercial preparations have between 0.5 and 2.0 calories/mL; most contain no milk (lactose) products. For patients who need fluid restriction, the higher concentrated formulas may be valuable, but they may cause diarrhea. Because of reduced kidney function with aging, some recommend that protein should contribute no more than 20% of the formula's total calories. If formula is sole source of nutrition, consider one that contains fiber (25 g/d is optimal).

Table 46. Examples of Lactose-Free Oral and Enteral Products							
Product	Kcal/mL	mOsm	Protein (g/L)	Water (mL/L)	Na (mEq/L)	K (mEq/L)	Fiber (g/L)
Oral—low residue							
Boost Basic	1.06	650	37.0	850	37.0	41.0	0
Boost Plus	1.50	670	61.0	780	37.0	38.0	< 1
Ensure	1.06	470	37.3	845	37.0	40.0	0
Ensure Plus	1.50	690	54.9	769	46.0	40.0	0
Nu Basics	1.00	480	35.0	842	38.0	32.0	0
Nu Basics Plus	1.50	620	42.4	776	50.8	48.0	0

(continues)

Product	Kcal/mL	mOsm	Protein (g/L)	Water (mL/L)	Na (mEq/L)	K (mEq/L)	Fiber (g/L)
Oral—clear liquid							
Citrisource	0.76	700	37.0	876	10.0	1.6	0
Resource	1.06	430	33.0	842	24.0	1.3	0
Diabetes formulations							
Choicedm TF	1.06	300	45.0	850	37.0	47.0	14.4
Glucerna	1.00	355	41.8	853	40.0	40.0	14.4
Enteral—low residue							
Isocal	1.06	270	34.0	850	23.0	34.0	0
Osmolite	1.06	300	37.2	841	28.0	26.0	0
Nutren 1.0	1.00	315	40.0	852	38.1	32.0	0
Enteral—low volume							
Deliver	2.00	640	75.0	710	35.0	43.0	0
Nutren 2.0	2.00	745	80.0	700	56.5	49.2	0
Enteral—high fiber							
Boost with Fiber	1.00	480	43.0	850	31.0	41.0	12.0
Ensure Fiber with FOS	1.06	—	36.0	780	37.0	40.0	12.0
Jevity	1.06	310	44.4	830	40.0	40.0	14.4
Ultracal	1.06	310	44.0	850	40.0	41.0	14.4
Nutren 1.0 with fiber	1.00	320	40.0	840	38.1	32.0	14.0

Table 46. Examples of Lactose-Free Oral and Enteral Products (cont.)

Important Drug-Enteral Interactions

- Soybean formulas increase fecal elimination of thyroxine; time administration of thyroxine and enteral nutrition as far apart as possible.
- Enteral feedings reduce absorption of phenytoin; administer phenytoin at least 2 h following a feeding and delay feeding at least 2 h after phenytoin is administered; monitor levels and adjust doses, as necessary.
- Check with pharmacy about suitability and best way to administer sustained-release, enteric-coated, and micro-encapsulated products (eg, omeprazole, lansoprazole, diltiazem, fluoxetine, verapamil).

Tips for Successful Tube Feeding

- Gastrostomy tube feeding may be either intermittent or continuous.
- Jejunostomy tube feedings must be continuous.
- Continuous tube feeding is associated with less frequent diarrhea but with higher rates of tube clogging.
- To prevent clogging and to provide additional free water, flushing with at least 30–60 cc of water 4–6 times a day is recommended. Sometimes sugar-free carbonated beverages, cranberry juice, or meat tenderizer can restore patency to clogged tubes.
- Diarrhea, which occurs in 5%–30% of persons receiving enteral feeding, may be related to the osmolality of the formula, the rate of delivery, high sorbitol content in liquid medications (eg, APAP, lithium, oxybutynin, furosemide), or other patient-related factors such as antibiotic use or impaired absorption.
- To help prevent aspiration, maintain a 30-degree elevation of the head of the bed during continuous feeding and for at least 2 h following bolus feedings.
- Do not administer bulk-forming laxatives (eg, methylcellulose or psyllium) through feeding tubes.

MALNUTRITION

• Check gastric residual volume before each bolus feeding and hold feeding for at least 1 h if residual is more than half of previous feeding volume. Metoclopramide (*Reglan*) 5–10 mg [5 mg/5 mL] qid may be useful for high gastric residual volume problems once mechanical obstruction has been excluded.

Parenteral Nutrition

Indicated in those with digestive dysfunction precluding enteral feeding. Delivers protein as amino acids, carbohydrate as dextrose, and fat as lipid emulsions.

Peripheral Parenteral Nutrition: For short-term use. Requires rotation of peripheral IV site every 72 h. Solution osmolarity of less than 900 mOsm/L is recommended to reduce risk of phlebitis (see **Table 47**).

Total Parenteral Nutrition: Must be administered through a central catheter, which may be inserted peripherally.

Table 47. Caloric Value and Osmolarity of Parenteral Solutions		
Resolution	Caloric Value (Kcal/L)	Osmolarity (mOsm/L)
Dextrose (%)		
5	170	250
10	340	500
20	680	1000
Lipid emulsions (%)		
10	1100	230
20	2200	330–340

Source: Bçikston SJ. In: Ewald GA, McKenzie CR. *Manual of Medical Therapeutics.* 28th ed. Boston: Little, Brown;1995:36. Copyright © 1995 by Little, Brown & Company. Reprinted with permission.

SHOULDER PAIN: DIFFERENTIAL DIAGNOSIS AND TREATMENT

Rotator Cuff Tendinitis, Subacromial Bursitis, or Rotator Tendon Impingement on Clavicle

Dull ache radiating to upper arm. Painful arc (on abduction 60–120 degrees and external rotation) is characteristic. Also can be distinguished by applying resistance against active range of motion while immobilizing the neck with hand.

Treatment: Identify and eliminate provocative, repetitive injury (eg, avoid overhead reaching). A brief period of rest and immobilization with a sling may be helpful. Pain control with APAP or NSAIDs (**Table 48**), home exercises or PT (especially assisted range of motion and wall walking), and corticosteroid injections may be useful.

Rotator Cuff Tears

Mild to complete; characterized by diminished shoulder movement. If severe, patients do not have full range of active or passive motion. The "drop arm" sign (the inability to maintain the arm in an abducted 90-degree position) indicates supraspinatus and infraspinatus tear. Weakness of external rotation (elbows flexed, thumbs up with examiner's hands outside patient's elbows; patient is asked to resist inward pressure) is common. MRI establishes diagnosis.

Treatment: If due to injury, a brief period of rest and immobilization with a sling may be helpful. Pain control with APAP or NSAIDs (**Table 48**), home exercises or PT (especially assisted range of motion and wall walking) may be useful. If no improvement after 6–8 wk of conservative measures, consider surgical repair.

Bicipital Tendinitis

Pain felt on anterior lateral aspect of shoulder, tenderness in the groove between greater and lesser tuberosities of the humerus. Pain is produced on resisted flexion of shoulder, flexion of the elbow, or supination (external rotation) of the hand and wrist with the elbow flexed at the side.

Treatment: Identify and eliminate provocative, repetitive activities (eg, avoid overhead reaching). A period of rest (at least 7 d with no lifting) and corticosteroid injections are major components of therapy. After rest period, PT should focus on stretching biceps tendon (eg, putting arm on doorframe and hyperextending shoulder, with some external rotation).

Frozen Shoulder (Adhesive Capsulitis)

Loss of passive external (lateral) rotation, abduction, and internal rotation of the shoulder to less than 90 degrees. Usually follows three phases: painful (freezing) phase lasting wks to a few mo; adhesive (stiffening) phase lasting 4–12 mo; resolution phase lasting 6–24 mo.

Treatment: Avoid rest and begin PT and home exercises for stretching the arm inflexion, horizontal adduction, and internal and external rotation. Corticosteroid injections may reduce pain and permit more aggressive PT. Consider surgical manipulation under anesthesia or arthroscopic dilation of capsule.

BACK PAIN: DIFFERENTIAL DIAGNOSIS AND TREATMENT

Acute Lumbar Strain (Low Back Pain Syndrome)

Acute pain frequently precipitated by heavy lifting or exercise. Pain may be central or more prominent on one side and may radiate to sacroiliac region and buttocks. Pain is aggravated by motion, standing, and prolonged sitting, and relieved by rest. Sciatic pain may be present even when neurologic examination is normal.

Treatment: Most can continue normal activities. If a patient obtains symptomatic relief from bed rest, generally 1–2 d lying in a semi-Fowler position or on side with the hips and knees flexed with pillow between legs will suffice. Treat muscle spasm with the application of ice, preferably in a massage over the muscles in spasm. APAP or NSAIDs (**Table 48**) can be used to control pain. As pain diminishes, encourage patient to begin isometric abdominal and lower-extremity exercises. Symptoms often recur. Education on back posture, lifting precautions, and abdominal muscle strengthening may help prevent recurrences.

Acute Disk Herniation

Over 90% of cases occur at L4–L5 or L5–S1 levels, resulting in unilateral impairment of ankle reflex, toe and ankle dorsiflexion, and pain (commonly sciatic) on straight leg raising (can be tested from sitting position by leg extension). Pain is acute in onset and varies considerably with changes in position.

Treatment: Initially same as acute lumbar strain (above). If unresponsive, administer epidural injection of a combination of a long-acting corticosteroid with an epidural anesthetic. Consider surgery if recurrence or persistence with neurologic signs beyond 6–8 wk after conservative treatment. The value of epidural injections and surgery for pain without neurologic signs is controversial. (See **Table 2** and **Table 3**.)

Osteoarthritis and Chronic Disk Degeneration

Characterized by aching pain aggravated by motion and relieved by rest. Occasionally, hypertrophic spurring in a facet joint may cause unilateral radiculopathy with sciatica.

Treatment: Identify and eliminate provocative activities. Education on back posture, lifting precautions, and abdominal muscle strengthening. APAP or NSAIDs (**Table 48**). Corticosteroid injections may be useful. Consider opioids and other pain treatment modalities for chronic refractory pain (see p 116).

Unstable Lumbar Spine

Severe, sudden, short-lasting, frequently recurrent pain often brought on by sudden, unguarded movements. Pain is reproduced upon moving from the flexed to the erect position. Pain is usually relieved by lying supine or on side. Impingement on nerve roots by spurs from facet joints or herniated disks can cause similar complaints, although symptoms in these conditions usually worsen as time passes. Symptoms can mimic disk herniation or degeneration, or osteoarthritis. Lumbar flexion x-rays can be diagnostic.

Lumbar Spinal Stenosis

Symptoms increase on spinal extension (eg, with prolonged standing, walking downhill, lying prone) and decrease with spinal flexion (eg, sitting, bending forward while walking, lying in the flexed position). Only symptom may be fatigue or pain in legs when walking (pseudo-claudication). May have immobility of lumbar spine, pain with straight leg raises, weakness of muscles innervated by L4 through S1 (see **Table 2**). Over 4 yr, 15% improve, 15% deteriorate, and 70% remain stable.

Treatment: APAP or NSAIDs (**Table 48**) and exercises to reduce lumbar lordosis are sometimes beneficial. Corticosteroid injections may be useful. Surgical intervention is more effective than conservative treatment in relieving moderate or severe symptoms; however, recurrence of pain several years after surgery is common.

Vertebral Compression Fracture
Immediate onset of severe pain; worse with sitting or standing; sometimes relieved by lying down.

Treatment: See Osteoporosis (p 112). Bed rest, analgesia, and mobilization as tolerated. Calcitonin may provide symptomatic improvement. May require hospitalization to control symptoms. Percutaneous vertebroplasty or kyphoplasty may be effective for pain relief in refractory cases, but clinical trial data are lacking.

Nonrheumatic Pain (eg, Tumors, Aneurysms)
Gradual onset, steadily expanding, often unrelated to position and not relieved by lying down. Night pain when lying down is characteristic. Upper motor neuron signs may be present. Involvement is usually in thoracic and upper lumbar spine.

HIP PAIN: DIFFERENTIAL DIAGNOSIS AND TREATMENT
Trochanteric Bursitis
Pain in lateral aspect of the hip that usually worsens when patient sits on a hard chair, lies on the affected side, or rises from a chair or bed; pain may improve with walking. Local tenderness over greater trochanter is often present, and pain is often reproduced on resisted abduction of the leg or internal rotation of the hip. However, trochanteric bursitis does not produce limited range of motion, pain on range of motion, pain in the groin, or radicular signs.

Treatment: Identify and eliminate provocative activities. Check for leg length discrepancy, prescribe orthotics if appropriate. Injection of a combination of a long-acting corticosteroid with an anesthetic is most effective treatment.

Osteoarthritis
"Boring" quality pain in the hip, often in the groin, and sometimes referred to the back or knee with stiffness after rest. Passive motion is restricted in all directions if disease is fairly advanced. In early disease, pain in the groin on internal rotation of the hip is characteristic.

Treatment: See Osteoarthritis (p 97). Elective total hip replacement is indicated for patients who have radiographic evidence of joint damage and moderate to severe persistent pain or disability, or both, that is not substantially relieved by an extended course of nonsurgical management.

National Institutes of Health Consensus Development Conference Statement September 12–14, 1994 (reviewed 1998).

Hip Fracture
Sudden onset, usually after a fall, with inability to walk or bear weight, frequently radiating to groin or knee.

Treatment: Treatment is surgical with open reduction and internal fixation, hemiarthroplasty, or total hip replacement, depending on site of fracture and amount of displacement. For patients who were nonambulatory prior to the fracture, conservative management is an option.

Nonrheumatic Pain
Referred pain from viscera, radicular pain from the lower spine, avascular necrosis, Paget's disease, metastasis.

OSTEOARTHRITIS
Nonpharmacologic Approaches
- Superficial heat: Hot packs, heating pads, paraffin, or hot water bottles (moist heat is better).
- Deep heat: Microwave, shortwave diathermy, or ultrasound.
- Biofeedback and transcutaneous electrical nerve stimulation.
- Exercise (especially water-based), PT, OT: Strengthening, stretching, range of motion, functional activities.
- Weight loss: Especially for low back, hip, and knee arthritis.
- Splinting: Avoid splinting for long periods of time (eg, > 6 wk) since periarticular muscle weakness and wasting may occur. Bracing (eg, neoprene sleeves over the knee) to correct malalignment is often helpful.
- Assistive devices: Cane should be used in the hand contralateral to the affected knee or hip.
- Surgical intervention (eg, debridement, meniscal repair, prosthetic joint replacement).

Pharmacologic Intervention (See also p 116.)
Topical Analgesics: Liniment, capsaicin cream.
Intra-articular Injections:
- Corticosteroids: May be particularly effective if monoarticular symptoms (eg, methylprednisolone acetate, triamcinolone acetonide, and triamcinolone hexacetonide) 20–40 mg for large joints (eg, knee, ankle, shoulder), 10–20 mg for wrists and elbows, and 5–15 mg for small joints of hands and feet; often mixed with lidocaine 1% or its equivalent (in equal volume with corticosteroids) for immediate relief.
- Hyaluronan: Sodium hyaluronate (*Hyalgan*) injections weekly for 5 wk or hylan G-F 20 (*Synvisc*) 3 injections 1 wk apart for knee osteoarthritis.
Initial Drug Treatment of Choice: APAP not to exceed 4 g/d (ACR) (see **Table 48**).
Nutriceuticals: glucosamine (500 mg 3x/d) or chondroitin (400 mg 3x/d), or both, have been effective for some patients. Combination tablets and timed-release formulations (1500 mg and 1200 mg, respectively) are available. Clinical trials in the United States are in process.
NSAIDs: Often provide pain relief but have higher rates of side effects (see **Table 48**). Misoprostol (*Cytotec*) 100–200 mg qid with food [T: 100, 200] or a proton-pump inhibitor (see **Table 29**) may be valuable prophylaxis against NSAID-induced ulcers in high-risk patients. Selective COX-2 inhibitors have lower likelihood of causing gastroduodenal ulcers than nonselective NSAIDs. All may increase INR in patients receiving warfarin.
Oral Analgesics: Eg, tramadol, other opioids (see **Table 58**).

Table 48. APAP and NSAIDs

Class, Drug	Usual Dosage for Arthritis	Formulations	Comments (Metabolism, Excretion)
APAP (*Tylenol*)	650 mg q 4–6 h	[T: 80, 325, 500, 650; C: 160, 325, 500; S: elixir 120/5 mL, 160/5 mL, 167/5 mL, 325/5 mL; S: 160/5 mL, 500/15 mL; Sp: 120, 325, 600]	Drug of choice for chronic musculoskeletal conditions; no anti-inflammatory properties; hepatotoxic above 4 g/d; at high doses ($\geq$ 2g/d) may increase INR in patients receiving warfarin; reduce dose 50%–75% if liver or kidney disease or if harmful or hazardous drinking (L, K)
Extended release (*Tylenol ER*)	1300 mg tid	[ER: 650]	
ASA	650 mg q 4–6 h	[T: 81, 325, 500, 650, 975; Sp: 120, 200, 300, 600]	(K)
Extended release (*Ext Release Bayer 8 Hour*,* ZORprin*)	1300 mg tid or 1600–3200 mg bid	[CR: 650, 800]	
Enteric-coated*	1000 mg qid	[T: 81, 162, 325, 500, 650, 975]	
Nonacetylated Salicylates			Do not inhibit platelet aggregation; fewer GI and renal side effects; no reaction in ASA-sensitive patients
Choline magnesium salicylate (*Tricosal, Trilisate*)	3 g/d in 1, 2, or 3 doses	[T: 500, 750, 1000; S: 500 mg/5mL]	(K)
Choline salicylate (*Arthropan*)	4.8–7.2 g/d divided	[S: 870 mg/5 mL]	(L, K)
Magnesium salicylate (eg, *Backache, Doan's, Mobigesic, Momentum*)	650 mg q 4 h, max 3600–4800/d in 3–4 divided doses; 1090 mg tid	[T: 325, 377, 580; C: 467]	Avoid in renal failure
Salsalate (eg, *Disalcid, Mono-Gesic, Salflex*)	1500 mg to 4 g/d in 2 or 3 doses	[T: 500, 750; C: 500]	(K)
Sodium salicylate* (*Uracel*)	325–650 mg q 4 h	[T: 325, 650]	

Table 48. APAP and NSAIDs (cont.)

Class, Drug	Usual Dosage for Arthritis	Formulations	Comments (Metabolism, Excretion)
Nonselective NSAIDs			
Diclofenac (*Cataflam, Voltaren, Voltaren-XR*)	50–150 mg/d in 2 or 3 doses	[T: 50, enteric coated 25, 50, 75, ER 100]	(L)
Extended release 50 mg with 200 μg misoprostol (*Arthrotec 50*) 75 mg with 200 μg misoprostol (*Arthrotec 75*)	100 mg/d	[T: 100]	(L)
Diflunisal (*Dolobid*)	500–1000 mg/d in 2 doses	[T: 250, 500]	(K)
Etodolac (*Lodine*)	200–400 mg tid–qid	[T: 400, 500; ER 400, 500, 600; C: 200, 300]	Fewer GI side effects (L)
Fenoprofen (*Nalfon*)	200–600 mg tid–qid	[C: 200, 300; T: 600]	Higher risk of GI side effects (L)
Flurbiprofen (*Ansaid*)	200–300 mg/d in 2, 3, or 4 doses	[T: 50, 100]	(L)
Ibuprofen (eg, *Advil, Motrin, Nuprin*)**	1200–3200 mg/d in 3 or 4 doses	[T: 100, 200, 300, 400, 600, 800; ChT: 50, 100; S: 100 mg/5 mL]	Fewer GI side effects (L)
Indomethacin (*Indochron, Indocin*)	25–50 mg bid–tid	[C: 25, 50; Sp: 50; S: 25 mg/5 mL; Inj]	High risk of GI side effects; increased risk of CNS side effects (L)
Extended release (*Indocin SR*)	75 mg/d or bid	[C: 75]	Increased risk of CNS side effects
Ketoprofen (*Actron, Orudis*)	50–75 mg tid	[T: 12.5; C: 25, 50, 75]	(L)
Sustained release (*Actron 200,** Oruvail*)	200 mg/d	[C: 100, 150, 200]	(L)
Ketorolac (*Toradol*)	10 mg q 4–6 h, 15 mg IM or IV q 6 h	[T: 10; Inj]	Duration of use should be limited to 5 d (K)
Meclofenamate sodium	200–400 mg/d in 3 or 4 doses	[C: 50, 100]	High incidence of diarrhea (L)
Meloxicam (*Mobic*)	7.5–15 mg/d	[T: 7.5, 15]	Has some COX-2 selectivity (L)
Nabumetone (*Relafen*)	500–1000 mg bid	[T: 500, 750]	Fewer GI side effects (L)
Naproxen (*Aleve,** Naprosyn*)	200–500 mg bid–tid	[T: 220, 275, 375, 500; S: 125 mg/5 mL]	(L)
Delayed release (*EC-Naprosyn*)	375–500 mg bid	[T: 375, 500]	(L)
Extended release (*Naprelan*)	750–1000 mg daily	[T: 375, 500, 750]	(L)

(*continues*)

Table 48. APAP and NSAIDs (cont.)			
Class, Drug	Usual Dosage for Arthritis	Formulations	Comments (Metabolism, Excretion)
Naproxen sodium (Anaprox)	275 mg or 550 mg bid	[T: 275, 550]	
Oxaprozin (Daypro)	1200 mg/d	[C: 600]	(L)
Piroxicam (Feldene)	10 mg/d	[T: 10, 20]	(L)
Sulindac (Clinoril)	150–200 mg bid	[T: 150, 200]	May have higher rate of renal impairment (L)
Tolmetin (Tolectin)	600–1800 mg/d in 3 or 4 doses	[T: 200, 600; C: 400]	(L)
Selective COX-2 Inhibitors			Less GI ulceration; do not inhibit platelets; may increase INR if taking warfarin; avoid if moderate or severe hepatic insufficiency; may induce renal impairment
Celecoxib (Celebrex)	100–200 mg bid	[C: 100, 200]	Contraindicated if allergic to sulfonamides
Rofecoxib (Vioxx)	12.5–25 once daily	[T: 12.5, 25, 50; S: 12.5 mg/5 mL, 25 mg/5 mL]	Contraindicated if allergic to sulfonamides
Valdecoxib (Bextra)	10 mg once/d	[T: 10, 20]	Contraindicated if allergic to sulfonamides

* Also available without prescription in a lower tablet strength.
** Available without a prescription.

GOUT
Definition
Urate crystal disease that may be expressed as acute gouty arthritis, usually in a single joint of foot, ankle, knee, or olecranon bursa; or chronic arthritis.

Precipitating Factors
- Alcohol, heavy ingestion
- Allopurinol, stopping or starting
- Binge eating
- Dehydration
- Diuretics
- Fasting
- Infection
- Serum uric acid levels, any change up or down
- Surgery

Evaluation of Acute Gouty Arthritis
Joint aspiration to remove crystals and microscopic examination to establish diagnosis; serum uric acid (can be normal during flare).

Management
Treatment of Acute Gouty Flare: Experts differ regarding order of choices:
- Intra-articular injections (see p 97)
- NSAIDs (see **Table 48**)
- Colchicine (more toxic in older persons; more effective if given within 24 hr of symptom onset)

- Oral 0.5–0.6 mg (1 tablet) q 1–2 h until symptoms abate, GI toxicity occurs, or maximum dose of 6 mg/24-h period has been given.
- IV 1–2 mg in 10–20 mL NS given over 3–5 min
  - may repeat the following day
  - contraindicated in patients who have had recent oral colchicine
  - avoid in patients with renal or hepatic disease
  - potential for severe bone marrow toxicity
- Prednisone 20–40 mg po qd until response, then rapid taper
- ACTH 75 IU SC or cosyntropin (*Cortrosyn*) 75 µg SC; may repeat daily for 3 d

Treatment of Hyperuricemia Following Acute Flare: Colchicine 0.5–0.6 mg/d for 2–4 wk prior to initiation of any treatment in **Table 49** and continued until serum uric acid has returned to normal.

Table 49. Medications Useful in Managing Chronic Gout			
Drug	Usual Dosage	Formulations	Comments (Metabolism, Excretion)
Allopurinol (*Zyloprim*)	100–200 mg qd	[T: 100, 300]	Do not initiate during flare; reduce dose in renal or hepatic impairment; increase dose by 100 mg every 2–4 wk to normalize serum urate level; monitor CBC; rash is common (K)
√ Colchicine	0.5–0.6 mg	[T: 0.5, 0.6; Inj]	Follow CBC (L)
Probenecid (*Benemid*)	500–1500 mg in 2–3 divided doses	[T: 500]	Adjust dose to normalize serum urate level or increase urine urate excretion; inhibits platelet function; may not be effective if renal impairment (K, L)
√ Sulfinpyrazone (*Anturane*)	50 mg po bid to 100 mg qid	[T: 100; C: 200]	Inhibits platelet function (K)

Note: √ = preferred for treating older persons.

PSEUDOGOUT
Definition
Crystal-induced arthritis (especially affecting wrists and knees) associated with calcium pyrophosphate.

Risk Factors
- Advanced osteoarthritis
- Diabetes mellitus
- Gout
- Hemochromatosis
- Hypercalcemia
- Hyperparathyroidism
- Hypomagnesemia
- Hypophosphatemia
- Hypothyroidism
- Neuropathic joints
- Older age

Precipitating Factors
- Acute illness
- Dehydration
- Minor trauma
- Surgery

Evaluation of Acute Arthritis

Joint aspiration and microscopic examination to establish diagnosis; x-ray indicating chondrocalcinosis (best seen in wrists, knees, shoulder, symphysis pubis).

Management of Acute Flare

See **Gout** (p 100). Colchicine is less effective in pseudogout.

POLYMYALGIA RHEUMATICA, GIANT CELL (TEMPORAL) ARTERITIS

Definitions

Polymyalgia Rheumatica (PMR): proximal limb and girdle stiffness without tenderness but with constitutional symptoms (eg, fatigue, malaise) and elevated sedimentation rate, often $\geq$ 100, and C-reactive protein (CRP); consider ultrasound.

Giant Cell (Temporal) Arteritis (GCA): medium to large vessel vasculitis that presents with symptoms of PMR, headache, scalp tenderness, jaw or tongue claudication, visual disturbances, TIA or stroke, elevated sedimentation rate, and CRP.

Diagnosis and Management

- PMR is a clinical diagnosis supported by an increased sedimentation rate. Management is low-dose (eg, 5–20 mg/d) prednisone or its equivalent. Some patients with milder symptoms may respond to NSAIDs alone. Follow symptoms and CRP or sedimentation rate. Maintain therapy for at least 1 yr to prevent relapse. Consider osteoporosis prevention medication (see p 112).
- GCA is confirmed by temporal artery biopsy, but treatment should not wait for pathologic diagnosis. Begin prednisone (1.0–1.5 mg/kg/d) or its equivalent while biopsy and pathology are pending. Consider adding methotrexate 10 mg orally per wk and folate 5 mg/d, which may have a steroid-sparing effect. After 2–4 wk, begin gradual taper to lowest dose that will control symptoms and CRP or sedimentation rate. Maintain therapy for at least 1 yr to prevent relapse. Consider osteoporosis prevention medication (see p 112).

NEUROLOGIC DISORDERS

TREMORS

Table 50. Classification of Tremors				
Type	Hz	Associated Conditions	Features	Treatment
Cerebellar	3–5	Cerebellar disease	Present only during movement; ↑ with intention; ↑ amplitude as target is approached	Symptomatic management
Essential	4–12	Familial in 50% of cases	Varying amplitude; common in upper extremities, head, neck; ↑ with antigravity movements, intention, stress, medications	Long-acting propranolol or atenolol (see p 32); or primidone (*Mysoline*) 100 mg qhs start, titrate to 0.5–1.0 g/d in 3–4 divided doses [T: 50, 250; S: 250 mg/5 mL]; or gabapentin (see p 108)
Parkinson's	3–7	Parkinson's disease, parkinsonism	"Pill rolling;" present at rest; ↑ with emotional stress or when examiner calls attention to it; commonly asymmetric	See Parkinson's disease (p 106)
Physiologic	8–12	Normal	Low amplitude; ↑ with stress, anxiety, emotional upset, lack of sleep, fatigue, toxins, medications	Treatment of exacerbating factor

DIZZINESS

Table 51. Classification of Dizziness				
Primary Symptom	Features	Duration	Diagnosis	Management
Dizziness	Lightheadedness 1–30 min after standing	Seconds to minutes (E)	Orthostatic hypotension	See p 61
	Impairment in > 1 of the following: vision, vestibular function, spinal proprioception, cerebellum, lower-extremity peripheral nerves	Occurs with ambulation (C)	Multiple sensory impairments	Correct or maximize sensory deficits; PT for balance and strength training

(continues)

Table 51. Classification of Dizziness (cont.)

Primary Symptom	Features	Duration	Diagnosis	Management
	Unsteady gait with short steps; ↑ reflexes and/or tone	Occurs with ambulation (C)	Ischemic cerebral disease	Aspirin; modification of vascular risk factors; PT
	Provoked by head or neck movement; reduced neck range of motion	Seconds to minutes (E)	Cervical spondylosis	Behavior modification; reduce cervical spasm and inflammation
Drop attacks	Provoked by head or neck movement, reduced vertebral artery flow seen on Doppler or angiography	Seconds to minutes (E)	Postural impingement of vertebral artery	Behavior modification
Vertigo	Brought on by position change, positive Dix-Hallpike test	Seconds to minutes (E)	Benign paroxysmal positional vertigo	Epley's maneuvers to reposition crystalline debris; exercises provoking symptoms may be of help
	Acute onset, nonpositional	Days	Labyrinthitis (vestibular neuronitis)	Meclizine (see p 67)
	Low-frequency sensorineural hearing loss and tinnitus	Minutes to hours (E)	Ménière's disease	Meclizine for acute symptom relief; diuretics and/or salt restriction for prophylaxis
	Vascular disease risk factors, cranial nerve abnormalities	10 min to several hours (E)	TIAs	Aspirin; modification of vascular risk factors

Note: C = chronic; E = episodic.
Source: Data from Colledge NR, Barr-Hamilton RM, Lewis SJ, et al. Evaluation of investigations to diagnose the causes of dizziness in elderly people: a community based controlled study. *BMJ.* 1996;313(7060):788–792.

MANAGEMENT OF ACUTE STROKE
Attempt to Diagnose Cause
Examination:
- Cardiac (murmurs, arrhythmias, enlargement)
- Neurologic (serial examinations)
- Optic fundi
- Vascular (carotids and other peripheral pulses)

Tests:
- ABG
- Brain imaging (CT is adequate)
- BUN
- CBC
- LFTs
- Creatinine
- ECG
- Electrolytes
- ESR

Transesophageal echocardiography is preferred over transthoracic echocardiography for detection of cardiogenic emboli. Carotid duplex and transcranial Doppler studies can detect carotid and vertebrobasilar embolic sources, respectively. Magnetic resonance angiography is indicated if one is considering emergent thrombolytic therapy to reverse stroke progression within 6 h of onset of symptoms (thrombolytic therapy is of unproven benefit in older adults).

Provide Supportive Care
- Control BP: Do not lower SBP if it is < 180; higher BP should be lowered *gently*; some experts recommend not lowering SBP unless it is > 200.
- Correct metabolic and hydration imbalances.
- Detect and treat coronary ischemia, CHF, arrhythmias.
- Monitor and treat for hypoxia and hyperthermia.
- Monitor for depression.
- Refer to rehabilitation when medically stable.

Halt or Reverse Progression
Acute Noncardioembolic Stroke or TIA: Use ASA, 325 mg/d (range 81–1300 mg/d) or low-dose SC heparin, or both. The benefit of emergent thrombolytic therapy is unproven in older adults and should be considered on a case-by-case basis.

Cardioembolic Stroke: Begin full-dose heparin or warfarin anticoagulation 48 h after symptom onset. (See also p 17.)

Progressing Stroke or Crescendo TIAs: Even though there is no evidence that anticoagulation improves outcomes, some clinicians recommend it in this situation; ASA would be more conservative therapy.

Hemorrhagic Stroke: Supportive care.

STROKE PREVENTION
Risk Factor Modification
- Stop smoking
- Reduce SBP (goal < 140 mm Hg)
- Lower serum LDL (goal < 100 mg/dL)
- Start anticoagulation or antiplatelet therapy for atrial fibrillation (see p 17)

Antiplatelet Therapy for Patients With Prior TIA or Stroke
- First line is ASA 81–325 mg qd.
- Clopidogrel (*Plavix*) 75 mg qd [T: 75] if intolerant to ASA or ASA failure.
- Ticlopidine (*Ticlid*) 250 mg bid [T: 250] requires regular blood monitoring.
- Addition of dipyridamole (*Persantine*) 200–400 mg/d in 3–4 divided doses [T: 25, 50, 75] to ASA may provide additional benefit, or can be tried in cases of ASA or clopidogrel failure. A combination form of ASA (25 mg) and long-acting dipyridamole (200 mg) (*Aggrenox*) 1 tablet bid is available.
- In the absence of atrial fibrillation, warfarin therapy is no more effective than ASA in preventing strokes.

Table 52. Treatment Options for Carotid Stenosis			
Presentation	% Stenosis	Preferred Rχ	Comments
Prior TIA or stroke	≥ 70	CE	CE superior to medical therapy only if patient is reasonable surgical risk and facility has track record of low complication rate for CE (<5%)
Prior TIA or stroke	50–69	CE or MM	Serial carotid Doppler testing may identify rapidly developing plaques
Prior TIA or stroke	< 50	MM	CE of no proven benefit in this situation
Asymptomatic	≥ 80	CE or MM	CE should be considered only for the most healthy
Asymptomatic	< 80	MM	CE of no proven benefit in this situation

Note: CE = carotid endarterectomy; MM = medical management.

PARKINSON'S DISEASE

Parkinson's Disease Diagnosis Requires:

Bradykinesia, eg,
- Slowness of initiation of voluntary movements (eg, glue-footedness during gait initiation)
- Reduced speed and amplitude of repetitive movements (eg, tapping index finger and thumb together)
- Difficulty switching from one motor program to another (eg, multiple steps to turn during gait testing)

and 1 or more of the following:
- Muscular rigidity (eg, cogwheeling)
- 4–6 Hz resting tremor
- Impaired righting reflex (eg, retropulsed during sternal nudge)

Nonpharmacologic Management

- Patient education is essential, and support groups are often helpful; see p 190 for telephone numbers, Web sites.
- Exercise program
- Surgical therapies can be considered for disabling symptoms refractory to medical therapy. Tremor can be improved by thalamotomy or thalamic stimulation (fewer side effects). Dyskinesias can be treated by pallidotomy or pallidal and subthalamic stimulation.

Table 53. Drugs for Parkinson's Disease			
Class, Drug	Initial Dosage	Formulations	Comments (Metabolism, Excretion)
Dopamine			
√ Levodopa-carbidopa* (*Sinemet*)	25/100 tid	[T: 10/100, 25/100, 25/250]	Mainstay of PD therapy; increase dose as needed; watch for GI side effects, orthostatic hypotension, confusion (L)
√ Sustained-release levodopa-carbidopa* (*Sinemet CR*)	1 tab bid or tid	[T: 25/100, 50/200]	Useful at daily dopamine requirement ≥ 300 mg; slower absorption than carbidopa-levodopa; can improve motor fluctuations (L)

Table 53. Drugs for Parkinson's Disease (cont.)

Class, Drug	Initial Dosage	Formulations	Comments (Metabolism, Excretion)
Dopamine agonists			More CNS side effects than dopamine
Bromocriptine (*Parlodel*)	1.25 mg bid	[T: 2.5; C: 5]	Titrate over 3–4 wk to effective dose (15–30 mg/d); very expensive (L)
Pergolide (*Permax*)	0.05 mg qd	[T: 0.05, 0.25, 1]	Titrate over 3–4 wk to effective dose (2–3 mg/d in 2–3 divided doses); very expensive (K)
√ Pramipexole* (*Mirapex*)	0.125 mg tid	[T: 0.125, 0.25, 0.5, 1, 1.5]	Titrate over 3–4 wk to effective dose (1.5–4.5 mg/d) (K)
√ Ropinirole* (*Requip*)	0.25 mg tid	[T: 0.25, 0.5, 1, 2, 5]	Titrate over 3–4 wk to effective dose (3–16 mg/d) (L)
Catechol *O*-methyl-transferase (COMT) inhibitor			
√ Tolcapone (*Tasmar*)	100 mg tid	[T: 100, 200]	Monitor LFT q 6 mo (L, K)
√ Entacapone (*Comtan*)	200 mg with each L-dopa dose	[T: 200]	Adjunctive therapy with L-dopa; watch for nausea, orthostatic hypotension (L)
Anticholinergics			
Benztropine (*Cogentin*)	0.5 mg po qd	[T: 0.5, 1, 2]	Can cause confusion and delirium; helpful for drooling (L, K)
Trihexyphenidyl (*Artane, Trihexy*)	1 mg qd	[T: 2, 5; S: 2 mg/5 mL]	Same as above (L, K)
Dopamine reuptake inhibitor			
Amantadine (*Symmetrel*)	100 mg qd–bid	[T: 100; C: 100; S: 50 mg/5 mL]	Useful in early and late PD; watch closely for CNS side effects; do not D/C abruptly (K)
MAO B inhibitor			
Selegiline (*Carbex, Eldepryl*)	5 mg bid qam & noon	[T: 5]	Symptomatic benefit; not proven to be neuroprotective; expensive (L, K)

Note: √ = preferred for treating older persons; * = first-line therapy; PD = Parkinson's disease.

SEIZURES
Classification
- Generalized: All areas of brain affected with alteration in consciousness.
- Partial: Focal brain area affected, not necessarily with alteration in consciousness; can progress to generalized type.

Evaluation, Assessment
Initial:
- History: Neurologic disorders, trauma, drug and alcohol use
- Physical examination: General, with careful neurologic
- Routine tests: BUN, calcium, CBC, creatinine, ECG, EEG, electrolytes, glucose, head CT, LFT, magnesium
- Tests as indicated: Head MRI, lumbar puncture, oxygen saturation, urine toxic or drug screen

Common Causes:
- Advanced dementia
- CNS infection
- Drug or alcohol withdrawal
- Idiopathic causes
- Metabolic disorders
- Prior stroke (most common)
- Toxins
- Trauma
- Tumor

Management
- Treat underlying causes.
- Institute antiepileptic therapy (see **Table 54**). Virtually all antiepileptics can cause sedation and ataxia.

Table 54. Antiepileptic Therapy in Elderly Patients				
Drug	**Dosage (mg)**	**Target Blood Level (μg/mL)**	**Formulations**	**Comments (Metabolism, Excretion)**
Carbamazepine (*Tegretol*) (*Tegretol XR*)	200–600 bid	4–12	[T: 200; ChT: 100; S: 100/5 mL] [T: 100, 200, 400; C: CR 200, 300]	Many drug interactions; mood stabilizer (L, K) (L,K)
Gabapentin (*Neurontin*)	300–600 tid	NA	[C: 100, 300, 400; T: 600, 800; S: 250/5 mL]	Used as adjunct to other agents; adjust dose on basis of CrCl (K)
Lamotrigine (*Lamictal*)	100–300 bid	2–4	[T: 25, 100, 150, 200]	Prolongs PR interval; when used with valproic acid, begin at 25 mg qd, titrate to 25–100 mg bid (L, K)
Levetiracetam (*Keppra*)	500–1500 q 12 h	NA	[T: 250, 500, 750]	Reduce dose in renal impairment: CrCl 30–50: 250–750 q 12 h CrCl 10–30: 250–750 q 12 h CrCl < 10: 500–1000 q 24 h
Oxcarbazepine (*Trileptal*)	300–1200 bid	NA	[T: 150, 300, 600; ChT: 2, 5, 25; S: 300/5 mL]	Can rarely cause hyponatremia (L)
Phenobarbital (*Luminal*)	30–60 bid–tid	20–40	[T: 15, 16, 30, 32, 60, 100; S: 20/5 mL]	Many drug interactions; not recommended for use in elderly patients (L)
Phenytoin (*Dilantin*)	200–300 qd	5–20*	[C: 30, 100; ChT: 50; S: 125/5 mL]	Many drug interactions; exhibits nonlinear pharmacokinetics (L)
Tiagabine (*Gabitril Filmtabs*)	2–12 bid–tid	NA	[T: 2, 4, 12, 16, 20]	Side-effect profile in elderly patients less well described (L)
Topiramate (*Topamax*)	25–100 qd–bid	NA	[T: 25, 100, 200; C: 15, 25]	May affect cognitive functioning at high doses (L, K)

Table 54. Antiepileptic Therapy in Elderly Patients (cont.)				
Drug	Dosage (mg)	Target Blood Level (μg/mL)	Formulations	Comments (Metabolism, Excretion)
Valproic acid (*Depacon*, *Depakene*, *Depakote*)	250–750 bid–tid	50–100	[T: ER 125, 250, 500; C: 125, 250; S: 250/5 mL]	Can cause weight gain; several drug interactions; mood stabilizer; follow LFTs and platelets; SR preparation (*Depakote ER*) also available [T: 500] (L)

Note: NA = not available.

* Phenytoin is extensively bound to plasma albumin. In cases of hypoalbuminemia or marked renal insufficiency, calculate adjusted phenytoin concentration (C):

$$C_{adjusted} = \frac{C_{observed} \ (\mu g/mL)}{0.2 \times albumin \ (g/dL) + 0.1.}$$

If creatinine clearance < 10 mL/min, use:

$$C_{adjusted} = \frac{C_{observed} \ (\mu g/mL)}{0.1 \times albumin \ (g/dL) + 0.1.}$$

Obtaining a free phenytoin level is an alternate method for monitoring phenytoin in cases of hypoalbuminemia or marked renal insufficiency.

APHASIA

Table 55. Aphasias In Which Repetition Is Impaired				
Type	Fluency	Auditory Comprehension	Associated Neurologic Deficits	Comments
Broca's	−	+	Right hemiparesis	Patient aware of deficit; high rate of associated depression; message board helpful for communication
Wernicke's	+	−	Often none	Patient frequently unaware of deficit; speech content usually unintelligible; therapy often focuses on visually based communication
Conduction	+	+	Occasional right facial weakness	Patient usually aware of the deficit; speech content usually intelligible
Global	−	−	Right hemiplegia with right field cut	Most commonly due to left middle cerebral artery thrombosis, which, if this is the cause, carries a poor prognosis for meaningful speech recovery

Figure 5. Algorithm for Diagnosis of Peripheral Neuropathy

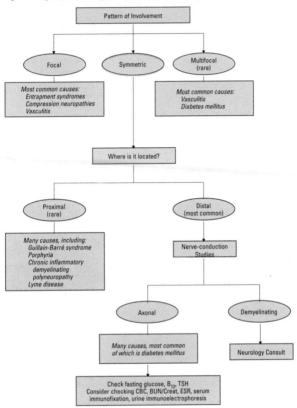

Source: Data from Poncelet AN. An algorithm for the evaluation of peripheral neuropathy. *Am Fam Phys.* 1998;57(4):755–764.

PERIPHERAL NEUROPATHY
Diagnosis See **Figure 5**.

Treatment
Prevention of Complications:
- Protect distal extremities from trauma—appropriate shoe size, daily foot inspections, good skin care, avoidance of barefoot walking.
- Maintain tight glycemic control in diabetic neuropathy.

Treatment of Painful Neuropathy: Start at low dose, increase as needed and tolerated:
- Nortriptyline (*Aventyl, Pamelor*) 10–100 mg qhs [T: 10, 25, 50, 75]; desipramine (*Norpramin*) 10–75 mg qam [T: 10, 25, 50, 75]
- Carbamazepine: (*Tegretol*) 200–400 mg tid [T: 200; ChT: 100; S: 100 mg/5 mL]; (*Tegretol XR*) 200 mg bid [T: 100, 200, 400; C: CR 200, 300]
- Gabapentin (*Neurontin*) 100–600 mg tid [C: 100, 300, 400; T: 600, 800; S: 250/5mL]
- Capsaicin cream (eg, *Zostrix*) 0.075% applied tid–qid [0.025%, 0.075%]
- Transcutaneous electrical nerve stimulation may be of benefit.
- Lidocaine 5% patches (*Lidoderm*) 1–3 patches covering the affected area up to 12 h/d [700 mg patch] is useful for post-herpetic neuralgia.

OSTEOPOROSIS

COMMONLY USED DEFINITIONS
- Established osteoporosis: occurrence of a minimal trauma fracture of any bone (WHO).
- Osteoporosis: a skeletal disorder characterized by compromised bone strength (bone density and bone quality) predisposing to an increased risk of fracture: NIH Consensus Development Panel. Osteoporosis prevention, diagnosis, and therapy. *JAMA* 2001; 285 (6):785–795.
- Osteoporosis: BMD 2.5 SD or more below that of younger normal individuals (T score) (WHO). Some experts prefer to use Z score, which compares an individual with a population adjusted for age, sex, and race.

RISK FACTORS FOR OSTEOPOROTIC FRACTURE
- Previous fracture as adult
- Dementia
- Depression
- Low calcium intake
- Low physical activity
- Fracture in 1st-degree relative
- Frailty
- Alcoholism
- Female sex
- Weight < 127 lb if female
- Cigarette smoking
- Early menopause
- Recurrent falls

TOXINS AND MEDICATIONS THAT CAN CAUSE OR AGGRAVATE OSTEOPOROSIS
- Alcohol (in excess)
- Anticonvulsants
- Corticosteroids
- Heparin
- Lithium
- Phenytoin
- Smoking
- Thyroxine (if overreplaced or in suppressive doses)

EVALUATION
Some experts recommend excluding secondary causes (serum PTH, TSH, calcium, phosphorus, albumin, alkaline phosphatase, bioavailable testosterone in men, renal and liver function tests, CBC, UA, electrolytes). Less consensus on: vitamin D levels, 24-h urinary calcium excretion; BMD test only if results could influence treatment or to establish baseline (see screening p 132). The value of monitoring BMD in persons already receiving treatment is unproven.

MANAGEMENT
Universal Recommendations
- Calcium 1200 mg/d
- Vitamin D 400–800 IU
- Avoid tobacco
- Weight-bearing exercise
- Falls prevention
- No more than moderate alcohol use

Pharmacologic Prevention
- Women over 70 with multiple risk factors are at high enough risk to initiate treatment without BMD testing.
- Some organizations have recommended initiating pharmacologic management in women with BMD T scores below –2 in the absence of risk factors and in women with T scores below –1.5 if other risk factors are present.

- Regimens:
  - Alendronate (*Fosamax*) 5 mg/d or 35 mg/wk [T: 5, 10, 35, 40, 70] (must be taken fasting with water; patient must remain upright and npo for at least 30 min after taking; relatively contraindicated in GERD) *or*
  - Risedronate (*Actonel*) 35 mg/wk or 5 mg/d [T: 5, 30, 35] (must be taken fasting or at least 2 h after evening meal; patient must remain upright and npo for 30 min after taking) *or*
  - Raloxifene (*Evista*) 60 mg/d [T: 60] *or*
  - Estrogen without progesterone (only women with hysterectomy) (see **Table 78** for dosing).

Pharmacologic Treatment
- Alendronate (*Fosamax*) 10 mg/d or 70 mg/wk [T: 5, 10, 35, 40, 70] (must be taken fasting with water; patient must remain upright and npo for at least 30 min after taking; relatively contraindicated in GERD) *or*
- Risedronate (*Actonel*) 35 mg/wk or 5 mg/d [T: 5, 30, 35] (must be taken fasting or at least 2 h after evening meal; patient must remain upright and npo for 30 min after taking) *or*
- Raloxifene (*Evista*) 60 mg/d [T: 60] *or*
- Calcitonin (*Calcimar, Cibacalcin, Miacalcin, Osteocalcin, Salmonine*) 100 IU/d SC [Inj: human (*Cibacalcin*) 0.5 mg/vial; salmon 200 units/mL) or 200 IU (*Miacalcin*) [200 units/activation] (intranasally, alternate nostrils every other day). May also be helpful for analgesic effect in patients with acute vertebral fracture (see also p 96) *or*
- Estrogen without progesterone (only women with hysterectomy) (see **Table 78** for dosing).
- Teriparatide (*Forteo*) 20 μg/d for up to 24 mo [Inj 3 mL, 28-dose disposable pen device] for high-risk patients; contraindicated in patients with Paget's disease or prior skeletal radiation therapy (L, K).

Table 56. Bone Outcomes and Level of Evidence* of Drugs for Osteoporosis				
Drug	Spine BMD and Fracture	Hip BMD	Hip Fracture	All Nonspinal Fractures
Estrogen**	improved–R	improved–R	reduced–R	no effect–R
Raloxifene	improved–R	improved–R	no data	no effect–R
Alendronate	improved–R	improved–R	reduced–R	reduced–R
Risedronate	improved–R	improved–R	reduced–R	reduced–R
Calcitonin (nasal)	improved–R	no effect–R	no effect–R	no effect–R

* The populations studied, sample sizes of individual studies, and duration of follow-up vary considerably; hence, this summary must be interpreted cautiously. Moreover, several randomized clinical trials are currently in progress and new findings may appear.
** The least expensive of the drugs listed.
Note: R = randomized clinical trial.

Table 57. Effects on Other Outcomes, Level of Evidence,* and Risks of Drugs for Osteoporosis						
Drug	CHD Risk Factors	CHD Prevention	CHD Treatment	Breast Cancer	Deep-Vein Thrombosis	Other
Estrogen	improved–R	↑ risk–R	no effect–R	↑ risk–R	↑ risk–R	↑ vaginal bleeding, stroke, PE ↓ colorectal cancer–R
Raloxifene	improved–R	↓ risk–R**	↓ risk–R	↓ risk–R	↑ risk–R	↑ hot flushes–R
Alendronate	no data	no data	no data	no data	no data	esophagitis
Risedronate	no data	no data	no data	no data	no data	
Calcitonin (nasal)	no data	no data	no data	no data	no data	rhinitis in 10%–12%

* The populations studied, sample sizes of individual studies, and duration of follow-up vary considerably; hence, this summary must be interpreted cautiously. Moreover, several randomized clinical trials are currently in progress and new findings may appear.
** Reduced risk demonstrated for high-risk women only.
Note: CHD = coronary heart disease; R = randomized clinical trial.

DEFINITION

An unpleasant sensory and emotional experience associated with actual or potential tissue damage

Acute Pain

Distinct onset, obvious pathology, short duration; common causes: surgery (postoperatively), headache

Chronic Pain

Persistent > 3 mo, often associated with functional and psychologic impairment, can fluctuate in character and intensity over time; common causes: arthritis, cancer, claudication, leg cramps, neuropathy, radiculopathy

EVALUATION

Key Points, Approach

- Assume patient's report is the most reliable evidence of pain intensity.
- Assess for pain on each presentation (older adults may be reluctant to report pain).
- Use synonyms for pain (eg, burning, aching, soreness, discomfort).
- Use a standard pain scale (see p 178); adapt for sensory impairments (eg, large print, written versus spoken).
- Assess cognitively impaired patients by:
  - Using simple tools or questions with yes/no answers.
  - Noting increased vocalizations (eg, moaning, groaning, crying).
  - Observing behaviors (eg, grimacing, irritability, failure to move an extremity, guarding).
  - Asking caregiver about recent changes in function, gait, behavior patterns, mood.
- Reassess regularly for improvement, deterioration, complications; keep log.
- Refer for comprehensive multidisciplinary evaluation for complex pain problem.

History and Physical

- Focus on a complete examination of pain source.
- Distinguish new illness from chronic condition.
- Analgesic history: effectiveness and side effects, current and previous prescription drugs, OTC drugs, "natural" remedies.
- Laboratory and diagnostic tests: to establish etiologic diagnosis.

Present Pain Complaint

Provocative (aggravating) and **P**alliative (relieving) factors
Quality (eg, burning, stabbing, dull, throbbing)
Region
Severity (eg, scale of 0 for no pain to 10 for worst pain possible; see p 178)
Timing (eg, when pain occurs, frequency and duration)

Psychosocial Assessment
Depression (see p 172 for screen), anxiety, mental status (see p 170 for screen).

Functional Assessment
ADLs, impact on activities (see pp 170,171 for screens) and quality of life.

Brief Pain Inventory
Use for comprehensive assessment of pain and its impact (see Appendixes, p 180).

PAIN MANAGEMENT
Acute Pain and Short-Term Management
• For severe pain, consider patient-controlled analgesic pump.
• Use fixed schedule of acetaminophen or opioids.
• Include nonpharmacologic strategies (eg, relaxation, heat or cold).

Chronic Pain
• Use multidisciplinary assessment and treatment.
• Educate patient for self-management and coping.
• Combine drug and nondrug strategies.
• Anticipate and attend to depression and anxiety.

Nonpharmacologic Treatment
• Educate patient and caregiver.
• Emphasize self-administered therapies (eg, heat, cold, massage, liniments and topical agents).
• Prescribe exercise, especially for chronic pain.
• Add therapy conducted by professionals (eg, distraction, relaxation techniques, music therapy, coping skills, biofeedback, imagery, hypnosis) as needed.
• When appropriate, obtain:
  - Rehabilitation medicine consult (OT, PT) for mechanical devices to minimize pain and facilitate activity (eg, splints), transcutaneous electrical nerve stimulation, range-of-motion and ADL programs.
  - Psychiatric pain management consult for somatization or hysteria, management of withdrawal.
  - Anesthesia pain management consult for possible interventional therapy (eg, neuroaxial analgesia, injection therapy, neuromodulation) when more conservative approaches are ineffective.

Pharmacologic Treatment
Selection of Agent(s):
• Base initial choice of analgesic on the severity and type of pain:
  - Consider nonopioids for mild pain (rating 0–3) (see **Table 48**).
  - Consider low-dose combination agents (see **Table 58**) for mild to moderate pain (rating 4–6) (eg, oxycodone, hydrocodone, tramadol with APAP).

- Consider potent and titratable mu opioid agonists (see **Table 58**) for more severe pain (rating 7–10) (eg, morphine, hydromorphone, oxymorphone).
- Consider adjuvant drugs (see **Table 59**) alone or in conjunction with opioids or nonopioids for neuropathic pain and other selected chronic conditions.
- Select lowest side-effect profile agents.
• Select least invasive route (usually oral) and fast-onset, short-acting analgesics for episodic or breakthrough pain.
• Use long-acting or sustained-release analgesics for continuous pain.
• Avoid long-term, nonselective NSAID use for chronic conditions.
• Consider COX-2 inhibitors for patients who would benefit from anti-inflammatory drug therapy on a continuous, long-term basis.
• Consider fixed-dose combinations (eg, APAP and hydrocodone or tramadol) for mild to moderate pain; do not exceed maximum dose for nonopioid.
• Avoid using multiple opioids or nonopioids when possible.
• Drugs with long half-life or depot effects (eg, methadone, levorphanol, transdermal fentanyl) need to be used and titrated cautiously, with close supervision of effects; duration of effect may exceed usual dose intervals because of reductions in metabolism and clearance.

Adjustment of Dosage:
• Begin with lowest dose possible, increasing slowly.
• Titrate dose on basis of persistent need for and use of medications for breakthrough pain. If using 3 or more doses of breakthrough pain medication per day, increase dose of sustained-release medication.
• Dose to therapeutic ceiling of nonopioid or NSAID if side effects permit.
• Increase opioid dose until pain relief achieved or side effects unmanageable before changing drugs (there is no maximum dose or analgesic ceiling with opioids).
• Use morphine equivalents as a common denominator for all dose conversions to avoid errors.
• When changing opioids, decrease equianalgesic dose by 25%–50% because of incomplete tolerance.
• Administer around-the-clock for continuous pain.
• Reassess, re-examine, and readjust therapy frequently until pain is relieved.

Management of Side Effects:
• Anticipate, prevent, and vigorously treat side effects; expect older patients to be more sensitive to side effects.
• Begin prophylactic laxative, osmotic, or stimulant when initiating opioid therapy (see **Table 31**); if patient taking sufficient fluids, cautiously increase fiber or psyllium; titrate laxative dose up with opiate dose. (See also p 65 stepped approach.)
• Monitor for sedation, delirium, urinary retention, constipation, respiratory depression, and nausea; tolerance develops to mild sedation, nausea, and impaired cognitive function.
• On long-term NSAID use, monitor periodically for GI blood loss, renal insufficiency, and other drug-drug and drug-disease interactions.
• Avoid the following drugs: carisoprodol, chlorzoxazone, cyclobenzaprine, indomethacin, meperidine, metaxalone, methocarbamol, nalbuphine, pentazocine, propoxyphene (see also p 187 for CMS criteria regarding inappropriate drug use).

Table 58. Opioid Analgesic Drugs				
Class, Drug	MS Equiv* (Route)	Starting Oral Dosage in Opioid-Naïve Patients	Formulations	Indication for Pain**
Short-Acting				
Codeine	200 mg (po)	15 mg q 4–6 h	[T: 15, 30, 60; S: 15/5 mL; Inj]	A
Codeine & APAP†	200 mg (po)	1–2 15/325 tabs q 4–6 h; if 1 tab used, add 325 mg APAP	[T: 15/325, 30/325, 60/325, 30/500, 30/650, 7.5/300, 15/300, 30/300, 60/300; S: 12/120/5 mL]	A
Hydrocodone & APAP† (eg, Lorcet, Lortab, Vicodin)	30 mg	5–10 mg q 4–6 h	[T: 10/325, 5/400, 7.5/400, 10/400, 2.5/500, 5/500, 7.5/500, 10/500, 7.5/650, 7.5/750, 10/650, 10/660; C: 5/500; S: 2.5/167/5 mL (contains 7% alcohol)	A
Hydrocodone & ASA (eg, Lortab ASA)	30 mg	5/500	[T: 5/500]	A
Hydrocodone & ibuprofen (eg, Vicoprofen)	30 mg	7.5/200	[T: 7.5/200]	A
Oxycodone (Oxy IR, Roxicodone)	20–30 mg (po)	5 mg q 3–4 h	[T: 5, 15, 30; C: 5; S: 5 mg/mL, 20 mg/mL]	A
Oxycodone & APAP† (Percocet, Tylox)	20 mg (po)	2.5–5 mg oxycodone q 6 h	[T: 2.5/325, 5/325, 5/500, 7.5/325, 7.5/500, 10/325, 10/650; C: 5/500; S: 5/325/5 mL]	A
Oxycodone & ASA (Percodan)	20 mg (po)	2.25–4.5 mg oxycodone q 6 h	[T: 2.25/325, 4.5/325]	A
Morphine (MSIR, Astramorph PF, Duramorph, Infumorph, Roxanol, OMS Concentrate, MS/L, RMS, MS/S)	30 mg (po), 10 mg (IV, IM, SC)	5 mg (po), 1–2 mg (IV) q 4–6 h	[C: 15, 30; soluble T: 15, 30; S: 10 mg/5 mL, 20 mg/5 mL, 100 mg/5 mL, 4 mg/mL, 20 mg/mL; Sp: 5, 10, 20, 30; Inj]	B
Hydromorphone (Dilaudid, Hydrostat)	7.5 mg (po), 1.5 mg (IV, IM, SC), 6 mg (rectal)	2 mg q 3–4 h	[T: 2, 4, 8; S: 5 mg/5 mL; Sp: 3; Inj]	B
Oxymorphone (Numorphan)	1 mg (IV, IM, SC), 10 mg (rectal)	0.5 mg IM, IV, SC q 4–6 h	[Sp: 5; Inj]	B

Table 58. Opioid Analgesic Drugs (cont.)				
Class, Drug	MS Equiv* (Route)	Starting Oral Dosage in Opioid-Naïve Patients	Formulations	Indication for Pain**
Fentanyl (*Actiq*)	NA	suck on 200 μg loz over 15 min, effect begins within 10 min	[loz on a stick: 200, 400, 600, 800, 1200, 1600 μg]	B
Tramadol (*Ultram*)	150–300 mg	25–50 mg q 4–6 h; not > 300 for age 75+	[T: 50]	B
Tramadol & APAP† (*Ultracet*)	37.5/325 mg	2 tabs po q 4–6 h pain; max 8 tabs/d‡	[T: 37.5/325]	B
Long-Acting				
ER Morphine (*MS Contin, Kadian*)	30 mg (po)	20–30 mg q 24 h, 15 mg q 12 h (*MS Contin* CR & XR tabs), 20 mg q 24 h (*Kadian* SR caps)	[T: CR 15, 30, 60, 100, 200, XR 15, 30, 60; C: SR 5, 20, 30, 60, 100]	B
ER Oxycodone (*OxyContin*)	20–30 mg (po)	20 mg q 24 h, 10 mg q 12 h	[T: CR 10, 20, 40, 80, 160]	B
Transdermal fentanyl (*Duragesic*)	NA (see package insert)	25 μg/h or higher (if able to tolerate 50 mg oral morphine equiv/ 24 h)	[25 μg/h (10 cm²), 50 μg/h (20 cm²), 75 μg/h (30 cm²), 100 μg/h (40 cm²)]	B

* MS Equiv = morphine sulphate (MS) equivalent dose: morphine equivalency = dose of opioid equivalent to 10 mg of parenteral morphine or 30 mg of oral morphine with chronic dosing. The parenteral: oral ratio is greater (1:6) during acute dosing, ie, 10 mg IM MS = 60 mg po MS. NA = not applicable.
** A = mild to moderate pain; B = moderate to severe pain.
† Caution: total APAP dose should not exceed 4 g/d.
‡ Treatment not to exceed 5 d; if CrCl < 30 mL/min, max is 2 tab q 12 h, not to exceed 5 d.

Table 59. Adjuvant Drugs for Pain Relief in Elderly Patients			
Class, Drug	Formulations	Starting Dosage	Comments
Antiarrhythmic			
Mexiletine (*Mexitil*)	[C: 150, 200, 250]	150 mg initial dose, increasing to 150 mg bid, then tid, then qid only if tolerated and no evidence of conduction block	Side effects such as tremor, dizziness, unsteadiness, paresthesias are common; rarely, hepatic damage and blood dyscrasias occur; avoid use in patients with preexisting heart disease; start with low dose and titrate slowly; recommend initial and follow-up ECGs; titrate to tid–qid dosing

(*continues*)

Table 59. Adjuvant Drugs for Pain Relief in Elderly Patients (cont.)			
Class, Drug	**Formulations**	**Starting Dosage**	**Comments**
Anticonvulsants (see Table 54)			If one does not work, try another
Antidepressants (see Table 22)			Use low-dose desipramine or nortryptiline; data on SSRIs lacking
Corticosteroids (see Table 25)			Low-dose medical management may be helpful in inflammatory conditions
Counterirritants			
Camphor-menthol-phenol (*Sarna*)*	[lot: camphor 5%, menthol 5%, phenol 5%]	prn	May be effective for arthritic pain, but effect limited when pain affects multiple joints; can cause skin injury, especially if used with heat or occlusive dressing
Camphor & phenol (*Campho-Phenique*)*	[S: camphor 5%, phenol 4.7%]	prn	
Methylsalicylate and menthol			
(*Ben-Gay* oint,* *Icy Hot* cre*)	[methylsalicylate 18.3%, menthol 16%]	3–4 × / d	Apply to affected area
(*Ben-Gay* extra strength cre*)	[methylsalicylate 30%, menthol 10%]	3–4 × / d	Apply to affected area
Trolamine salicylate (*Aspercreme* rub*)	[trolamine salicylate 10%]	≤ 4 × / d	Apply to affected area
Other agents			
Baclofen (*Lioresal*)	[T: 10, 20; Inj]	2.5–5 mg bid–tid	Probably increased sensitivity and decreased clearance; monitor for weakness, urinary dysfunction; avoid abrupt discontinuation because of CNS irritability
Capsaicin (eg, *Capsin, Capzasin, No Pain-HP, R-Gel, Zostrix*)	[cre, lot, gel, roll-on: 0.025%, 0.075%]	3–4 × / d	Renders skin and joints insensitive by depleting and preventing reaccumulation of substance P in peripheral sensory neurons; may cause burning sensation; instruct patient to wash hands after application to prevent eye contact; do not apply to open or broken skin

* Available OTC.

Note: Various adjuvant classes are useful for the treatment of neuropathic pain. TCAs are often helpful for migraine or tension headaches and arthritic conditions. Baclofen is particularly useful for muscle-related problems, such as spasms.

PALLIATIVE AND END-OF-LIFE CARE

DEFINITION
"The active total care of patients, controlling pain and minimizing emotional, social and spiritual problems at a time when disease is not responsive to active treatment" (WHO, 1990).

PRINCIPLES
- Support, educate, and treat both patient and family.
- Address physical, psychologic, social, and spiritual needs.
- Use multidisciplinary team (physicians, nurses, social workers, chaplain, pharmacist, physical and occupational therapists, dietitian, family and caregivers, volunteers).
- Focus on symptom management, comfort, meeting goals, completion of "life business," healing relationships, and bereavement.
- Make care available 24 h/d, 7 d/wk.
- Offer bereavement support.
- Supply therapeutic environment (palliation can be given in any location).
- Provide for all dying patients.

QUALITY OF LIFE
Ways to help patient and family enhance quality of life at the end of life:
- Communicate, listen
- Teach stress management, coping
- Use all available resources
- Support decision making
- Encourage conflict resolution
- Help complete unfinished business
- Urge focus on non-illness-related affairs
- Urge a focus on one day at a time
- Help anticipate grief, losses
- Help focus on attainable goals
- Encourage spiritual practices
- Promote physical, psychologic comfort

END-OF-LIFE DECISIONS
Follow principles involved in informed decision making (see **Figure 2**).

Hospice Referral
- Patients, families, or other health care provides can refer, but a physician's order is required for admission to a hospice program.
- Referral is appropriate when curative treatment is no longer indicated (ie, ineffective, too burdensome side effects) and life is limited to months.
- Hospice must be accepted by the patient or family, or both, and can be rescinded at any time.
- Hospice provides palliative medications, durable medical supplies and equipment, team member visits as needed and desired by patient and family (physician, nurses, home health aide, social worker, chaplain) and volunteer services.
- Optimal hospice care requires adequate time in the program; referral when death is imminent does not take full advantage of hospice care.
- Hospice care is usually delivered in patient's home, but it can be delivered in a nursing home or residential care facility (long-term care, assisted living) or in an inpatient setting (hospice-specific or contracted facility) if acuity or social circumstances warrant.

Advance Directives

Designed to respect patient's autonomy and determine his/her wishes about future life-sustaining medical treatment if unable to indicate wishes.

Oral Statements

- Conversations with relatives, friends, clinicians are most common form; should be thoroughly documented in medical record for later reference.
- Properly verified oral statements carry same ethical and legal weight as those recorded in writing.

Instructional Advance Directives (DNR Orders, Living Wills)

- Written instructions regarding the initiation, continuation, withholding, or withdrawal of particular forms of life-sustaining medical treatment.
- May be revoked or altered at any time by the patient.
- Clinicians who comply with such directives are provided legal immunity for such actions.

Durable Power of Attorney for Health Care or Health Care Proxy

A written document that enables a capable person to appoint someone else to make future medical treatment choices for him or her in the event of decisional incapacity (see **Figure 2**).

Key Interventions, Treatment Decisions to Include in Advance Directives:

- Resuscitation procedures
- Mechanical respiration
- Chemotherapy, radiation therapy
- Dialysis
- Simple diagnostic tests
- Pain control
- Blood products, transfusions
- Intentional deep sedation

Withholding or Withdrawing Therapy

- There is no ethical or legal difference between withholding an intervention (not starting it) and withdrawing life-sustaining medical treatment (stopping it after it has been started).
- Beginning a treatment does not preclude stopping it later; a time-limited trial may be appropriate.
- Palliative care should not be limited, even if life-sustaining treatments are withdrawn or withheld.
- Decisions on artificial feeding should be based on the same criteria applied to ventilators and other medical treatment.

Euthanasia

- Active euthanasia: direct intervention, such as lethal injection, intended to hasten a patient's death; a criminal act of homicide.
- Passive euthanasia: withdrawal or withholding of unwanted or unduly burdensome life-sustaining treatment; appropriate in certain circumstances.
- Assisted suicide: the patient's intentional, willful ending of his/her own life with the assistance of another; a criminal offense in most states.

MANAGEMENT OF COMMON END-OF-LIFE SYMPTOMS

Pain

- The most distressing symptom for patients and caregivers.

- If intent is to relieve suffering, the risk that sufficient medication will produce an unintended effect (hastening death) is morally acceptable.
- Primary goal: to alleviate suffering at end of life. See Pain (p 115) for assessment and interventions.
- Alternate routes may be needed, eg, transdermal, transmucosal, rectal, vaginal, topical, epidural, and intrathecal.
- Recommend expert pain management consult if pain not adequately relieved with standard analgesic guidelines and interventions.
- Additional treatment may include:
  - radionuclides and bisphosphonates (for metastatic bone pain).
  - treatments (eg, radiotherapy, chemotherapy) directed at source of pain.
- Pain crisis: Sedation at end of life for intractable pain and suffering is an important option to discuss with patients. Ketamine (*Ketalar*) 0.1 mg/kg IV bolus. Repeat as needed q 5 min. Follow with infusion of 0.015 mg/kg/min IV (SC if IV access not available at 0.3–0.5 mg/kg). Decrease opioid dose by 50%. Benzodiazepine may be useful. Observe for problems with increased secretions and treat (see section on excessive secretions, p 124).

Weakness, Fatigue
Nonpharmacologic:
- Modify environment to decrease energy expenditure (eg, placement of phone, bedside commode, and drinks).
- Adjust room temperature to patient's comfort.
- Teach energy-conserving techniques (eg, reordering tasks—eating first, resting, then bathing).
- Modify daily procedures (eg, sitting while showering, not standing).
Pharmacologic:
- Treat remediable causes such as pain, medication toxicity, insomnia, anemia, and depression.
- Consider psychostimulants (eg, dextroamphetamine [*Dexedrine*] 2.5 mg po qam or bid *or* methylphenidate [*Ritalin*] 5–10 mg po qam or bid); monitor for signs of psychosis, agitation, or sleep disturbance.

Dysphagia
Nonpharmacologic:
- Feed small, frequent amounts of pureed or soft foods.
- Avoid spicy, salty, acidic, sticky, and extremely hot or cold foods.
- Keep head of bed elevated for 30 min after eating.
- Instruct patient to wear dentures and to chew thoroughly.
- Use suction machine when necessary.
Pharmacologic:
- For painful mucositis: 1:2:8 mixture of diphenhydramine elixir: lidocaine [2%–4%]: *Maalox* as a swish-and-swallow suspension before meals.
- For candidiasis: clotrimazole 10 mg troches, 5 doses/d, *or* fluconazole 150 mg po followed by 100 mg po qd × 5 d.
- For severe halitosis: antimicrobial mouthwash; fastidious oral and dental care; treat putative respiratory tract infection with broad-spectrum antibiotics.

Dyspnea
Nonpharmacologic:
- Teach positions to facilitate breathing, elevate head of bed.
- Teach relaxation techniques.
- Eliminate smoke and allergens.
- Assure brisk air circulation (facial breeze) with a room fan; oxygen is indicated only for symptomatic hypoxemia (ie, $SaO_2 < 90\%$ with pulse oximetry).

Pharmacologic:
- Opioids: oral morphine conc (20 mg/mL): 1/4 to 1/2 mL sl/po; repeat in 10–15 min prn); nebulized morphine 2.5 mg in 2–4 cc NS *or* fentanyl 25–50 μg in 2–4 cc NS; *or* IV morphine 1 mg or equivalent opioid q 5–10 min.
- Bronchodilators (see **Table 70**).
- Diuretics, if evidence of volume overload (see **Table 16**).
- Anxiolytics (eg, lorazepam po/sl/SC 0.5–2 mg q 2–4 h or prn); titrate slowly to effect.

Constipation
Most common cause: side effects of opioids, medications with anticholinergic side-effects (see **Table 31**). Use stimulant or osmotic laxative.

Bowel Obstruction
Indications for Radiographic Evaluation:
- To differentiate constipation and mechanical obstruction
- To confirm the obstruction, determine site and nature if surgery is being considered

Nonpharmacologic Management:
- Nasogastric intubation: only if surgery is being considered, for high-level obstructions, and poor response to pharmacotherapy
- Percutaneous venting gastrostomy: for high-level obstructions and profuse vomiting not responsive to antiemetics
- Palliative surgery
- Hydration: IV or hypodermoclysis

Pharmacologic Management (aimed at specific symptoms):
- Nausea and vomiting: haloperidol (*Haldol*) po, IM 0.5–5 mg ($\leq$ 10 mg) q 4–8 h prn; ondansetron (*Zofran*) IV (over 2–5 min) 4 mg q 12 h, po 8 mg q 12 h (L) [Inj; T: 4, 8, 24; S: 4 mg/5 mL], but costly; see also **Table 32**.
- Spasm, pain, and vomiting: scopolamine IM, IV, SC 0.3–0.65 mg q 4–6 h prn; oral 0.4–0.8 mg q 4–8 h prn; transdermal 2.5 cm^2 patch applied behind the ear q 3 d (L) [Inj; T: 0.4; patch 1.5 mg] or hyoscyamine (*Levsin/SL*) sublingual [T: 0.125; S: 0.125 mg/mL] 0.125–0.25 tid–qid.
- Diarrhea and excessive secretions: loperamide (*Imodium A-D*) see **Table 33**; octreotide (*Sandostatin*) SC 0.15–0.3 mg q 12 h (L) [Inj], very expensive.
- Pain: see **Table 58**.
- Inflammation due to malignant obstruction: dexamethasone (*Decadron*) oral: 4 mg qid × 5–7 d.

Excessive Secretions
Nonpharmacologic: Positioning and suctioning, as needed
Pharmacologic: Glycopyrrolate 0.1–0.4 mg IV/SC q 4 h prn *or* scopolomine 0.3–0.6 mg SC prn *or* transdermal scopolomine patch q 72 h *or* atropine 0.3–0.5 mg SC, sublingual, nebulized q 4 h prn

Cough See Respiratory Diseases (p 143).

Nausea, Vomiting See Gastrointestinal Diseases (p 66).

Malnutrition, Dehydration See also Malnutrition (p 90).
Nonpharmacologic:
- Educate patient and family on effects of disease progression resulting in lack of appetite and weight loss.
- Promote interest, enjoyment in meals (eg, alcoholic beverage if desired, involve patient in meal planning, small frequent feedings, cold or semi-frozen nutritional drinks).
- Good oral care is important.

Pharmacologic:
- Corticosteroids: Dexamethasone 1–2 mg po tid; methylprednisolone 1–2 mg po bid; prednisone 5 mg po tid.
- Hormone therapy: Megestrol acetate 200–800 mg qd.

Altered Mental Status, Delirium See Delirium (p 39).

Anxiety, Depression
- Provide opportunity to discuss feelings, fears, existential concerns
- Referral to appropriate team members (spiritual, nursing)
- Medicate (see Anxiety, p 21, and Depression, p 46).

Source: Fine P. *Hospice Companion—Processes to Optimize Care During the Last Phase of Life.* 2d ed. Scottsdale, AZ: VistaCare, Inc.; 2000.

PREOPERATIVE CARE
Cardiac Risk Assessment

Figure 6. Reducing Cardiac Risk in Noncardiac Surgery

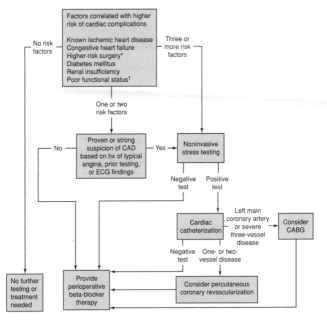

* Intraperitoneal, intrathoracic, or suprainguinal vascular procedures
† Inability to walk 4 blocks or climb 2 flights of stairs

Source: Adapted with permission from Fleisher LA, Eagle KA: Lowering cardiac risk in noncardiac surgery. *N Engl J Med* 2001; 345:1677–1682. Copyright © 2001, Massachusetts Medical Society. All rights reserved.

Pulmonary Risk Assessment

Assessing the patient for risk of pulmonary complications (respiratory failure, pneumonia, atelectasis) includes the following risk factors:

Smoking: To lower risk, patients should quit at least 8 wk prior to surgery.

COPD: Bronchodilators, physical therapy, antibiotics, and corticosteroids given preoperatively can reduce risk.
ASA Class: III—severe systemic disease; IV—life-threatening systemic disease; V—moribund.
Surgical Site: Upper abdominal, thoracic, > 3-h surgeries pose the greatest increased risk.
Note: Routine spirometry has not been shown to be useful in risk assessment.

Other Assessments
Anticoagulation Status: See pp 17–20.
Cognitive Status: Unrecognized dementia is a risk factor for postoperative delirium. Measure preoperative cognitive status with Mini-Cog (see p 170) or MMSE.
Nutritional Status: Poor nutritional status can impair wound healing. Measure height, weight, serum albumin.
Routine Laboratory Tests: Recommended: Hemoglobin and hematocrit, electrolytes, creatinine, BUN, ECG, CXR, albumin. Optional: CBC, platelets, ABG, PT, PTT.
Cataract Surgery: Routine laboratory testing or cardiopulmonary risk assessment is unneccessary for cataract surgery performed under local anesthesia.
Advance Directives: Establish or update.

PERIOPERATIVE MANAGEMENT
β-Blocker Use
For patients at risk for cardiac complications (see **Figure 6**), begin β-blocker agent (eg, atenolol or bisoprolol) orally 1–2 wk prior to surgery to achieve heart rate < 70 beats/min. Continue therapy until 2 wk after surgery, with a goal of < 80 beats/min in the postoperative period. Withhold β-blockers if heart rate is < 55 beats/min; SBP < 100; or the patient has asthma, decompensated CHF, or third degree heart block.

Endocarditis Prophylaxis
Depends on cardiac condition and type of procedure (see pp 132–134).

DVT Prophylaxis (see also pp 17–20)
General Surgery: LDUH, 5000 units SC 2 h before surgery and q 12 h after surgery, or LMWH (enoxaparin [*Lovenox*] 30 mg SC q 12 h postoperatively); and elastic stockings and/or IPC devices for higher risk patients.
Total Hip Replacement: LMWH, low-molecular-weight heparinoid or warfarin (begin 12 h before or 12–24 h after surgery; adjust INR 2.0 to 3.0) or dose-adjusted heparin
Total Knee Replacement: LMWH or factor Xa inhibitor or warfarin or IPC
Surgical Hip Fracture Repair: IPC plus either LMWH or warfarin

Common Problems to Monitor
- Confusion: see p 39
- Intra- and postoperative coronary events: postoperative ECG to check
- Malnutrition: see p 90
- Pain: see p 115
- Polypharmacy: review medications daily
- Pulmonary complications: minimized by incentive spirometry, coughing, early ambulation
- Rehabilitation: encourage early mobility
- Skin breakdown: see p 128

PRESSURE ULCERS

DEFINITION
Any lesion caused by unrelieved pressure resulting in damage of underlying tissue; usually occurs over bony prominence.

ETIOLOGIC FACTORS FOR PRESSURE ULCER DEVELOPMENT
- Pressure
- Shear
- Friction

INTRINSIC RISK FACTORS
- Immobility (eg, chairbound)
- ↑ Age
- Malnutrition
- Moisture (eg, incontinence)
- ↓ Sensory perception

EVALUATION
- Screen for presence of intrinsic risk factors (see above).
- Determine intensity of risk status using validated tool, eg, Braden Scale; see Braden BJ, Bergstrom N. Clinical utility of the Braden Scale for predicting pressure sore risk. *Decubitus* 1989;2(3):44–51; for online versions of the scale: http://www.skinwound.com/online_training_manual/braden_scale.htm (for a downloadable PDF file) http://text.nlm.nih.gov (in AHRQ pressure ulcer practice guideline).
- Assess skin daily, especially persons with one or more risk factors.
- Determine level of tissue injury by using staging criteria:
  - **Stage I:** An observable pressure-related alteration of intact skin whose indicators as compared with an adjacent or opposite area on the body may include changes in one or more of the following: skin temperature (warmth or coolness), tissue consistency (firm or boggy feel), and/or sensation (pain, itching). The ulcer appears as a defined area of persistent redness in lightly pigmented skin, whereas in darker skin tones, it may appear with persistent red, blue, or purple hues.
  - **Stage II:** Partial-thickness skin loss involving epidermis and/or dermis; presents as abrasion, blister, or shallow crater.
  - **Stage III:** Full-thickness skin loss involving damage or necrosis of subcutaneous tissue which may extend down to, but not through, underlying fascia; presents as deep crater with or without undermining of adjacent tissue.
  - **Stage IV:** Full-thickness skin loss with extensive destruction, tissue necrosis, or damage to muscle, bone, or supporting structures. May have associated undermining of sinus tracts. Note: eschar-covered ulcers cannot be staged until eschar is removed.
- Absence of signs of healing over 2-wk period should result in complete reassessment of factors that affect healing and of wound management strategies.
- Heel ulcers: Without signs of infection or inflammation, do not debride dry eschar. With signs of infection or inflammation or wet eschar, surgically debride; initiate antibiotic therapy; obtain vascular consult.

PREVENTION AND MANAGEMENT

Protect Wound and Surrounding Skin from Further Trauma
- Employ pressure-reduction strategies:
  - Reposition every 1–2 h.
  - Use pressure-reducing or relieving cushions, mattresses, and heel protectors.
  - Avoid doughnut cushions.
  - Avoid massaging reddened bony prominences.
- Reduce friction and shear:
  - Maintain head of bed elevation < 30 degrees.
  - Use lift sheet to reposition.

Promote Clean Wound Bed, Prevent Infection
- Debride necrotic tissue, eschar:
  - Sharp: scissors, forceps, scalpel
  - Mechanical: wet-to-dry dressings
  - Autolytic: moisture-retentive dressings or hydrogels
  - Chemical: topical enzymes (eg, *Accuzyme, Santyl*)

Autolytic methods or topical enzymes may be used in conjunction with sharp debridement to facilitate more rapid removal of necrotic tissue.
- Cleansing:
  - Cleanse with each dressing change and as needed.
  - Use normal saline.
  - Irrigate using 8 mm Hg pressure (19-gauge IV catheter and 35-cc syringe) when wound is deep, tunneled, or undermined.

Maintain Moist Wound Environment
- Use moisture-retentive dressings:
  - Calcium alginate
  - Continuous moist saline gauze
  - Foams
  - Hydrogel
  - Hydrocolloids
  - Transparent films

Eliminate Dead Space
- Pack dead space (tunnels, undermining):
  - Moistened saline gauze dressings or strips
  - Calcium alginate dressings

Control Exudate
- Use exudate-absorbing dressings:
  - Calcium alginate dressings
  - Foam dressings
  - Moistened saline gauze dressings

Diagnose and Treat Infection
- Signs of infection:
  - Nonhealing wound despite optimal treatment
  - Foul odor to exudate
  - Friable granulation tissue
  - Wound breakdown
  - Increasing pain
  - Edema
  - Serous exudate with concurrent inflammation
  - Peri-wound heat, erythema

- Swab culture is of limited value in diagnosing infection due to contaminated wound bed.
- Treatment of infection:
  - Remove necrotic tissue and purulent exudate from wound.
  - Use systemic antibiotics only in presence of spreading cellulitis, sepsis, or osteomyelitis.

Consider 2-wk trial of topical antibiotic for clean ulcers that are not healing or are continuing to produce exudate after 2–4 wk optimal care; antibiotic should be effective against gram-negative, gram-positive, and anaerobic organisms.

Support Healing Systemically
- Provide nutritional support (see p 90):
  - Increase calories and protein, including nutritional supplements as needed.
  - Obtain nutritional consult.
  - Use vitamin and mineral supplements.
- Provide adequate hydration with oral or parenteral fluids.

Surgical Repair
- Candidates: Stage IV pressure ulcers; severely undermined or tunneled wounds; ability to tolerate surgical procedure

Topical Wound Products

| Table 60. Wound and Pressure Ulcer Products, by Drainage and Stage | | | | | | | |
Product	Light	Drainage Moderate	Heavy	I	Wound Stage II	III	IV
Transparent film	X				X		
Foam island	X	X			X	X	
Hydrocolloids	X	X			X	X	
Petroleum-based nonadherent	X				X	X	
Alginate		X	X			X	X
Hydrogel	X				X	X	X
Gauze packing (moistened with saline)		X	X			X	X

| Table 61. Common Dressings for Pressure Ulcer Treatment | | | |
Dressing	Indications	Contraindications	Examples
Transparent film	Stage I ulcer Protection from friction Superficial scrape Autolytic debridement of slough Apply skin prep to intact skin to protect from adhesive	Draining ulcers Suspicion of skin infection or fungus	*Bioclusive* *Tegaderm* *Op-site*
Foam island	Stage II, III Low to moderate exudate Can apply as window to secure transparent film	Excessive exudate Dry, crusted wound	*Alleyn* *Lyofoam*

Table 61. Common Dressings for Pressure Ulcer Treatment (cont.)			
Dressing	**Indications**	**Contraindications**	**Examples**

Hydrocolloids	Stage II, III
	Low to moderate drainage
	Good peri-wound skin integrity
	Autolytic debridement of slough
	Left in place 3–5 d
	Can apply as window to secure
	  transparent film
	Can apply over alginate to
	  control drainage
	Must control maceration
	Apply skin prep to intact skin to
	  protect from adhesive
		Poor skin integrity
		Infected ulcers
		Wound needs packing
			DuoDerm
			Extra thin film
			  DuoDerm
			Tegasorb
			RepliCare
			Comfed

Alginate	Stage II, III, IV
	Excessive drainage
	Apply dressing within wound
	  borders
	Requires secondary dressing
	Must use skin prep
	Must control for maceration
		Dry or minimally
		  draining wound
		Superficial wounds
		  with maceration
			Sorbsan
			Kaltostat
			Algosteril
			AlgiDerm

Hydrogel
(amorphous
  gels)
	Stage II, III, IV
	Needs to be combined with
	  gauze dressing
	Stays moist longer than saline
	  gauze
	Changed 1–2 times/d
	Used as alternative to saline
	  gauze for packing deep
	  wounds with tunnels,
	  undermining
	Reduces adherence of gauze to
	  wound
	Must control for maceration
		Macerated areas
		Wounds with excess
		  exudate
			IntraSite gel
			Solosite gel
			Restore gel

(gel sheet)	Stage II
	Skin tears
	Needs to be held in place with
	  topper dressing
		Macerated areas
		Wounds with moderate
		  to heavy exudate
			Vigilon
			Restore
			Impregnated
			  Gauze

Gauze packing
(moistened
  with saline)
	Stage III, IV
	Wounds with depth, especially
	  those with tunnels,
	  undermining
	Must be remoistened often to
	  maintain moist wound
	  environment
			Square 2 × 2s,
			  4 × 4s
			Fluffed Kerlix
			Plain Nugauze

Source: Copyright © 1999 by Rita Frantz. Used with permission.

PREVENTION

PREVENTIVE TESTS AND PROCEDURES

Table 62. Recommended Primary and Secondary Disease Prevention for Persons Aged 65 and Over

Preventive Strategy	Frequency
USPSTF* Recommendations for Primary Prevention	
Bone densitometry (women)	at least once after age 65
BP screening	yearly
Influenza immunization	yearly
Lipid disorder screening	every 5 yr, more often in CAD, diabetes mellitus, peripheral arterial disease, prior stroke
Obesity (height and weight)	yearly
Pneumonia immunization	once at age 65**
Smoking cessation	at every office visit
Tetanus immunization	every 10 yr
USPSTF* Recommendations for Secondary Prevention	
FOBT and/or sigmoidoscopy	yearly/every 3–5 yr
Hearing impairment screening	yearly
Mammography, clinical breast examination***	every 1–2 yr
Pap smear†	at least every 3 yr
Visual impairment screening	yearly
Other‡ Recommendations for Primary Prevention	
Aspirin to prevent MI	daily
Diabetes mellitus screening	yearly
Other‡ Recommendations for Secondary Prevention	
Skin examination	yearly
Breast self-examination	monthly
Cognitive impairment screening	yearly
Colonoscopy (instead of sigmoidoscopy)	every 10 yr
PSA and digital rectal examination	yearly
TSH in women	yearly

* US Preventive Services Task Force. See http://www.ahrq.gov/clinic/uspstfix.htm
** Consider repeating pneumoncoccal vaccine every 6–7 yr.
*** Mammograms to age 70 are virtually universally recommended; many organizations, including the USPSTF, recommend that mammography should be continued in women over 70 who have a reasonable life expectancy.
† Pap smear testing can be stopped in most women after age 65. See p 167.
‡ Not endorsed by USPSTF for all older adults, but recommended in selected patients or by other professional organizations.

ENDOCARDITIS PROPHYLAXIS (AHA GUIDELINES)
Antibiotic Regimens Recommended (see Table 63)

Cardiac Conditions Requiring Prophylaxis
High-Risk Category: Prosthetic heart valves, previous endocarditis, surgical systemic pulmonary shunts

Moderate-Risk Category: Acquired valvular dysfunction (eg, rheumatic heart disease), hypertrophic cardiomyopathy, mitral valve prolapse with valvular regurgitation and/or thickened leaflets, most congenital heart malformations

Procedures Warranting Prophylaxis
Dental: Extractions, periodontal procedures, implants and reimplants, root canals, subgingival placement of antibiotic fibers or strips, initial placement of orthodontic bands but not brackets, intraligamentary local anesthetic injections, teeth cleaning where bleeding is expected
Respiratory Tract: Tonsillectomy and/or adenoidectomy, rigid bronchoscopy, surgery involving respiratory mucosa
GI Tract: Esophageal varices sclerotherapy, esophageal stricture dilation, endoscopic retrograde cholangiography with biliary obstruction, biliary tract surgery, surgery involving intestinal mucosa
GU Tract: Prostatic surgery, cystoscopy, urethral dilation

Cardiac Conditions Not Requiring Prophylaxis
Previous CABG surgery; mitral valve prolapse without valvular regurgitation; physiologic, functional, or innocent heart murmurs; previous rheumatic fever without valvular dysfunction; cardiac pacemakers; implanted defibrillators; isolated secundum atrial septal defect; surgical repair of atrial or ventricular septal defect

Procedures Not Warranting Prophylaxis
Dental: Restorative dentistry, local anesthetic injections, intracanal endodontic treatment, rubber dam placement, suture removal, placement of removable prosthodontic or orthodontic appliances, oral impressions, fluoride treatments, oral radiographs, orthodontic appliance adjustment
Respiratory Tract: Endotracheal intubation, flexible bronchoscopy (prophylaxis optional for high-risk patients), ear tube insertion
GI Tract: Transesophageal echocardiography, endoscopy (prophylaxis optional for high-risk patients)
GU Tract: Vaginal hysterectomy (prophylaxis optional for high-risk patients), urethral catheterization of uninfected tissue
Other: Cardiac catheterization, balloon angioplasty

Table 63. Endocarditis Prophylaxis Regimens	
Situation	**Regimen**
Dental, oral, respiratory tract, or esophageal procedures	
Standard general prophylaxis	Amoxicillin 2.0 g po 1 h before procedure
Unable to take oral medications	Ampicillin 2.0 g IM or IV $\leq$ 30 min before procedure
Allergic to penicillin	Clindamycin 600 mg or cephalexin 2.0 g or cefadroxil 2.0 g or azithromycin 500 mg or clarithromycin 500 mg po 1 h before procedure
Allergic to penicillin and unable to take oral medications	Clindamycin 600 mg or cefazolin 1.0 g IM or IV $\leq$ 30 min before procedure

(*continues*)

Table 63. Endocarditis Prophylaxis Regimens (cont.)	
Situation	**Regimen**
GU or GI procedures	
High-risk patients	Ampicillin 2.0 g IM or IV + 1 gentamicin 1.5 mg/kg IV or IM (not to exceed 120 mg) ≤ 30 min before procedure; 6 h later, ampicillin 1.0 g IM or IV or amoxicillin 1.0 g po
High-risk patients allergic to ampicillin or amoxicillin	Vancomycin 1.0 g IV over 1–2 h + gentamicin 1.5 mg/kg IV or IM (not to exceed 120 mg); complete injection or infusion ≤ 30 min before procedure
Moderate-risk patients	Amoxicillin 2.0 g po 1 h before procedure or ampicillin 2.0 g IM or IV ≤ 30 min before procedure
Moderate-risk patients allergic to ampicillin or amoxicillin	Vancomycin 1.0 g IV over 1–2 h, complete infusion ≤ 30 min before procedure

Note: See **Table 45** for details about antibiotics.
Source: Dajani AS, Taubert KA, Wilson W, et al. Prevention of bacterial endocarditis: Recommendations by the American Heart Association. *JAMA*. 1997;277:1794–1801. Copyright 1997, American Medical Association. Reprinted with permission.

Prophylaxis for Dental Patients with Total Joint Replacements (TJR)
Conditions Requiring: Inflammatory arthropathies (eg, rheumatoid arthritis, systemic lupus erythematosus); disease-, drug-, or radiation-induced immunosuppression; type 1 diabetes mellitus; first 2 yr following joint replacement; previous prosthetic joint infection; malnourishment; hemophilia
Conditions Not Requiring: Patients > 2 yr post-TJR who do not have one of the above conditions; patients with pins, plates, or screws
Dental Procedures Warranting: see those listed on p 133 for endocarditis
Suggested Prophylactic Regimens: (all given 1 h before procedure)
• Not allergic to penicillin: Amoxicillin, cephalexin, or cephradine 2.0 g po
• Not allergic to penicillin and unable to take oral medications: Ampicillin 2.0 g or cefazolin 1.0 g IM or IV
• Allergic to penicillin: Clindamycin 600 mg po
• Allergic to penicillin and unable to take oral medications: Clindamycin 600 mg IV

Source: Modified from American Dental Association and American Academy of Orthopaedic Surgeons. Antibiotic prophylaxis for dental patients with total joint replacements. *JADA*. 1997;128(7):1004–1007. Copyright © 1997 American Dental Association. Adapted 2002 with permission of ADA Publishing, a Division of ADA Business Enterprises, Inc.

EXERCISE PRESCRIPTION
Before Giving an Exercise Prescription
Screen patient for:
• Musculoskeletal problems: Decreased flexibility, muscular rigidity, weakness, pain, ill-fitting shoes
• Cardiac disease: Consider stress test if patient is beginning a vigorous exercise program and is sedentary with ≥ 2 cardiac risk factors (male gender, hypertension, smoking, diabetes mellitus, dyslipidemia, obesity, family hx, sedentary life style).

Individualize the Prescription

Specify short- and long-term goals; include the following components:

Flexibility: Static stretching; daily, > 15 sec per muscle group

Endurance: Walking, cycling, swimming at 50%–75% of maximum HR (220 – age for men; 220 – [0.6 × age] for women); 3–4 ×/wk; goal of 20–30 min duration

Strength: Muscle resistance (weight training); 3 sets (8–15 repetitions) per muscle group 2–3 ×/wk

Balance: Tai Chi, dance, postural awareness; 1–3 ×/wk

Patient Information: See http:// www.nia.nih.gov/exercisebook/

PSYCHOTIC DISORDERS

DIAGNOSIS
Differential Diagnosis
- Bipolar affective disorder
- Delirium
- Dementia
- Drugs: eg, antiparkinsonian agents, anticholinergics, benzodiazepines or alcohol (including withdrawal), stimulants, corticosteroids, cardiac drugs (eg, digitalis), opioid analgesics
- Late-life delusional (paranoid) disorder
- Major depression
- Physical disorders: hypo- or hyperglycemia, hypo- or hyperthyroidism, sodium or potassium imbalance, Cushing's syndrome, Parkinson's disease, B_{12} deficiency, sleep deprivation, AIDS
- Pain, untreated
- Schizophrenia
- Structural brain lesions: tumor or stroke
- Seizure disorder: eg, temporal lobe

Risk Factors for Psychotic Symptoms in Elderly Persons
Chronic bed rest, cognitive impairment, female gender, sensory impairment, social isolation

MANAGEMENT
- Alleviate underlying physical causes.
- Address identifiable psychosocial triggers.
- If psychotic symptoms are severe, frightening, or may affect safety, use antipsychotic.
- Olanzapine, quetiapine, risperidone are first choice because of fewer side effects (TD extremely high in elderly patients taking typical antipsychotics).

Table 64. Representative Antipsychotic Medications			
Class, Agent	Dosage*	Formulations	Comments (Metabolism)
Atypical Antipsychotics			
Aripiprazole (*Abilify*)	10–15 (1) initially; max 30/d	[T: 10, 15, 20, 30]	Very limited geriatrics experience; potential for somnolence; wait 2 wk between dose changes (CYP2D6, 3A4) (L)
Clozapine (*Clozaril*)	25–150 (1)	[T: 25, 100]	May be useful for parkinsonism and TD; sedation, orthostasis, anticholinergic, agranulocytosis, weight gain (L)
√ Olanzapine (*Zyprexa*)	2.5–10 (1)	[T: 2.5, 5, 7.5, 10, 15, 20; disintegrating tab: 5, 10, 15, 20]	Sedation, anticholinergic effects at high doses, weight gain, hyperglycemia, risk of diabetes; dose-related EPS (L)

Table 64. Representative Antipsychotic Medications (cont.)

Class, Agent	Dosage*	Formulations	Comments (Metabolism)
√ Quetiapine (*Seroquel*)	25–800 (1–2)	[T: 25, 100, 200, 300]	Sedation, orthostasis, no dose-related EPS (L, K)
√ Risperidone (*Risperdal*)	0.5–1 (1–2)	[T: 0.25, 0.50, 1, 2, 3, 4 scored; S: 1 mg/mL]	Orthostasis, dose-related EPS; do not exceed 6 mg (L, K)
Ziprasidone (*Geodon*)	20–80 (1–2)	[C: 20, 40, 60, 80]	May increase QT$_c$; very limited geriatric data (L)
Low Potency			
Thioridazine (eg, *Mellaril*)	25–200 (1–3)	[T: 10, 15, 25, 50, 100, 150, 200; S: 30 mg/mL]	Anticholinergic, orthostasis, QT$_c$ prolongation, sedation, TD; for acute use only (L, K)
Intermediate Potency			
Loxapine (*Loxitane*)	2.5–20 (1–3)	[C: 5, 10, 25, 50; S: 25 mg/mL]	Anticholinergic, orthostasis, sedation, TD; for acute use only (L, K)
High Potency			
Haloperidol (*Haldol*)	0.5–2 (1–3); depot 100–200 mg IM q 4 wk	[T: 0.5, 1, 2, 5, 10, 20; S: conc 2 mg/mL; Inj]	EPS, TD; for acute use only (L, K)

* Total mg/d (frequency/d).
Note: √ = preferred for treating older persons.

Table 65. Management of Side Effects of Antipsychotic Medications

Side Effect	Treatment	Comment
Drug-induced parkinsonism	Lower dose or switch to atypical antipsychotic	Often dose related
Akathisia (motor restlessness)	Switch to atypical antipsychotic, β-blocker (eg, propranolol [*Inderal*] 20–40 mg/d) or low-dose benzodiazepine (eg, lorazepam 0.5 mg bid)	Also seen with atypical antipsychotics; more likely with traditional agents
Hypotension	Slow titration; reduce dose; change drug class	More common with low-potency agents
Sedation	Reduce dose; give at bedtime; change drug class	More common with low-potency agents
TD	Stop drug (if possible); change to atypical antipsychotic	Increased risk in elderly; may be irreversible

Note: Periodic (q 4 mo) reevaluation of antipsychotic dose and ongoing need is important (see OBRA Regulations, p 184). Older persons are particularly sensitive to side effects of antipsychotic drugs. They are also at higher risk of developing TD. Periodic use of a side-effect scale such as the AIMS (see p 176) is highly recommended.

RENAL AND PROSTATE DISORDERS

ACUTE RENAL FAILURE
Definition
An acute deterioration in renal function defined by decreased urine output or increased values of renal function tests, or both

Precipitating and Aggravating Factors
- Acute tubular necrosis due to hypoperfusion or nephrotoxins
- Medications (eg, aminoglycosides, radiocontrast materials, NSAIDs, ACE inhibitors)
- Multiple myeloma
- Obstruction (eg, BPH)
- Vascular disease (thromboembolic, atheroembolic)
- Volume depletion or redistribution of extracellular fluid (eg, cirrhosis, burns)

Evaluation
- Review medication list
- Catheterize bladder, determine postvoid residual
- Determine fractional excretion of sodium (FENa):
- Perform UA
- Perform renal ultrasonography

$$FENa = \frac{urine\ Na/plasma\ Na \times 100\%}{urine\ creatinine/plasma\ creatinine}$$

(*FENa < 1% indicates prerenal cause; FENa > 3% indicates acute tubular necrosis; FENa 1%–3% is nondiagnostic. Note that some older persons who have prerenal cause may have FENa ≥ 1% because of age-related changes in sodium excretion.*)

Treatment
- D/C medications that are possible precipitants; avoid contrast dyes.
- If prerenal pattern, treat CHF if present (see p 27). Otherwise, volume repletion. Begin with fluid challenge 500–1000 cc over 30–60 min. If no response, give furosemide 100–400 mg IV.
- If obstructed, leave bladder catheter in place while evaluation and specific treatment are being implemented.
- If acute tubular necrosis, monitor weights daily, record intake and output, and monitor electrolytes frequently. Fluid replacement should be equal to urinary output plus other drainage plus 500 cc/d for insensible losses.
- Dialysis is indicated when severe hyperkalemia, acidosis, or volume overload cannot be managed with other therapies or when uremic symptoms (eg, pericarditis, coagulopathy, or encephalopathy) are present.

VOLUME DEPLETION (DEHYDRATION)
Definition
Losses of sodium and water that may be isotonic (eg, loss of blood) or hypotonic (eg, nasogastric suctioning)

Precipitating Factors
- Blood loss
- Diuretics
- GI losses
- Renal or adrenal disease (eg, renal sodium wasting)
- Sequestration of fluid (eg, ileus, burns, peritonitis)
- Age-related changes (impaired thirst, sodium wasting due to hyporeninemic hypoaldosteronism, and free water wasting due to renal insensitivity to antidiuretic hormone)

Evaluation
Clinical symptoms:
- Anorexia
- Nausea and vomiting
- Orthostatic lightheadedness
- Delirium
- Weakness

Clinical signs:
- Dry tongue and axillae oliguria
- Orthostatic hypotension
- Elevated heart rate
- Weight loss

Laboratory Tests
- Serum electrolytes
- Urine sodium (usually < 10 mEq/L) and FENa (usually < 1% but may be higher because of age-related sodium wasting)
- Serum BUN and creatinine (BUN/creatinine ratio often > 20)

Management
- Daily weight; monitor fluid losses and serum electrolytes, BUN, creatinine
- If mild, oral rehydration of 2–4 L of water/d and 4–8 g Na diet; if poor po intake, give IV D5W1/2 NS with potassium as needed
- If hemodynamically stable, give IV 0.9% saline 500 cc bolus and 200 cc/h until systolic BP ≥ 100 and no longer orthostatic. Then switch to D5W1/2 NS. Monitor closely in patients with a hx of CHF.

HYPERNATREMIA
Causes
- Pure water loss:
  - insensible losses due to sweating and respiration
  - central (eg, post-traumatic, CNS tumors, meningitis) diabetes insipidus or nephrogenic (eg, hypercalcemia, lithium) diabetes insipidus
- Hypotonic sodium loss:
  - renal causes: osmotic diuresis (eg, due to hyperglycemia); postobstructive diuresis; polyuric phase of acute tubular necrosis
  - GI causes: vomiting and diarrhea, nasogastric drainage, osmotic cathartic agents (eg, lactulose)
- Hypertonic sodium gain (eg, treatment with hypertonic saline)
- Impaired thirst (eg, delirious or intubated) or access to water (eg, functionally dependent) may sustain hypernatremia

Evaluation
- Measure intake and output.
- Obtain urine osmolality:
  - \> 800 mOsm/kg suggests extrarenal (if urine Na < 25 mEq/L) or remote renal water loss or administration of hypertonic Na^+ salt solutions (if urine Na > 100 mEq/L).
  - < 250 mOsm/kg and polyuria suggests diabetes insipidus.

Treatment
- Treat underlying causes.
- Correct slowly over at least 48–72 h using oral (can use pure water), nasogastric (can use pure water), or IV (D5W, 1/2 or 1/4 NS) fluids; correct at rate of no more than 1 mmol/L/h if acute (eg, developing over hours) and at no more than 10 mmol/L/d if of longer duration.
- Correct with normal saline only in cases of severe volume depletion with hemodynamic compromise; once stable, switch to hypotonic solution.
- When repleting, use the following formula to estimate the effect of 1 L of any infusate on serum Na:

$$\text{Change in serum Na} = \frac{\text{infusate Na} - \text{serum Na}}{\text{total body water} + 1}.$$

- Infusate Na (mmol/L): D5W = 0; 1/4 NS = 34; 1/2 NS = 77; NS = 154.
- Calculate total body water as a fraction of body weight (0.5 kg in older men and 0.45 kg in older women).
- Divide treatment goal (usually 10 mmol/L/d) by change in serum Na/L (from formula) to determine amount of solution to be given over 24 h.
- Compensate for any ongoing obligatory fluid losses, which are usually 1.0–1.5 L/d.
- Divide amount of solution for repletion plus amount for obligatory fluid losses by 24 to determine rate per h.

HYPONATREMIA
Causes
- With increased plasma osmolality: Hyperglycemia (1.6 mEq/L decrement for each 100 mg/dL increase in plasma glucose)
- With normal plasma osmolality (pseudohyponatremia): Severe hyperlipidemia, hyperproteinemia (eg, multiple myeloma)
- With decreased plasma osmolality:
  - With extracellular fluid (ECF) excess: Renal failure, heart failure, hepatic cirrhosis, nephrotic syndrome
  - With decreased ECF volume: Renal losses from salt-losing nephropathies, diuretics, osmotic diuresis, extrarenal loss due to vomiting, diarrhea, skin losses, and third-spacing (usually urine Na < 20 mEq/L, FENa < 1%, and uric acid > 4 mg/dL)
  - With normal ECF volume: Primary polydipsia (urine osmolarity < 100 mOsm/kg), hypothyroidism, adrenal insufficiency, SIADH (urine Na > 40 mEq/L and uric acid < 4 mg/dL)

Management

Only if symptomatic (eg, altered mental status, seizures) or severe acute hyponatremia (eg, < 120 mEq/L):

- Goal is 0.5 mEq/L/h rise in Na (more rapid correction can result in central pontine myelinolysis); time (in hours) to correct = (140 − Na)/0.5 mEq/L/h.
- Calculate free water excess (liters) = (0.5 × current body weight in kg) × (1 − [Na/140]).
- Target rate of free water removal (L/h) = free water excess/time to correct.
- Replace urine output with 3% saline or isotonic saline.
- Monitor Na closely and taper treatment when > 120 or symptoms resolve.

SIADH
Definition

Hypotonic hyponatremia (< 280 mOsm/kg) with:

- Less than maximally dilute urine (usually > 100 mOsm/kg)
- Elevated urine sodium (usually > 40 mEq/L)
- Normal volume status
- Normal renal, adrenal, and thyroid function

Precipitating Factors, Causes

- Drugs (eg, SSRIs, venlafaxine, chlorpropamide, carbamazepine, NSAIDs, barbiturates)
- Neuropsychiatric factors (eg, neoplasm, subarachnoid hemorrhage, psychosis, meningitis)
- Postoperative state, especially if pain or nausea
- Pulmonary disease (eg, pneumonia, tuberculosis, acute asthma)
- Tumors (eg, lung, pancreas, thymus)

Evaluation

- BUN, creatinine, serum cortisol, TSH
- CXR
- Review of medications
- Neurologic tests as indicated
- Urine sodium and osmolality

Management

Acute Treatment: See hyponatremia management (above)

Chronic Treatment:

- D/C offending drug or treat precipitating illness.
- Restrict water to 1000–1500 mL/d.
- Liberalize salt intake.
- Demeclocycline (*Declomycin*) 150–300 mg bid [T: 150, 300] (may be nephrotoxic in patients with liver disease).

BENIGN PROSTATIC HYPERPLASIA
Evaluation

Detailed medical hx focusing on the urinary tract physical examination, including a digital rectal examination and a focused neurologic examination; UA; measurement of serum creatinine. Measurement of PSA is optional.

Management

Mild Symptoms: (eg, AUA score ≤ 7; see p 183) watchful waiting

Moderate to Severe Symptoms: (eg, AUA score ≥ 8; see p 183) medical or surgical treatment

Medical Treatment:

- α-Blockers:
  - Terazosin (*Hytrin*) advance as tolerated—days 1–3, 1 mg/d hs; days 4–7, 2 mg; days 8–14, 5 mg; day 15 and beyond, 10 mg [T: 1, 2, 5, 10]
  - Doxazosin (*Cardura*) start 0.5 mg with max of 16 mg/d [T: 1, 2, 4, 8]
  - Prazosin (*Minipress*) start 1 mg/d (first dose hs) or bid with max 20 mg/d [T: 1, 2, 5]
  - Tamsulosin (*Flomax*) 0.4 mg half-hour after the same meal each day and increase to 0.8 mg if no response in 2–4 wk [T: 0.4]
- 5-α Reductase inhibitors:
  - Finasteride (*Proscar*) 5 mg/d [T: 5]
  - Dutasteride (*Avodart*) 0.5 mg/d [C: 0.5]

Surgical Management: Indicated if recurrent UTI, recurrent or persistent gross hematuria, bladder stones, or renal insufficiency are clearly secondary to BPH or as indicated by symptoms, patient preference, or failure of medical treatment. Options are:

- Transurethral resection of the prostate (TURP).
- Transurethral incision of the prostate (TUIP), which is limited to prostates whose estimated resected tissue weight (if done by TURP) would be 30 g or less.
- Open prostatectomy for large glands.

Source: McConnell JD, Barry MJ, Bruskewitz RC, et al. *Benign Prostatic Hyperplasia: Diagnosis and Treatment.* Clinical Practice Guideline No. 8. Rockville, MD: Agency for Health Care Policy and Research, Public Health Service, US Dept. of Health and Human Services, February 1994. AHCPR Publication No. 94-0582.

PROSTATE CANCER (see p 74)

ALLERGIC RHINITIS
Definition
- The most common atopic disorder.
- Symptoms include rhinorrhea; sneezing; and irritated eyes, nose, and mucous membranes.
- May be seasonal, but in older people is more often perennial.
- Postnasal drip, mainly from chronic rhinitis, is the most common cause of chronic cough.

Therapy
Nonpharmacologic: Avoid allergens, eliminate pets and their dander, dehumidify to reduce molds; reduce outdoor exposures during pollen season; reduce house dust mites by encasing pillows and mattresses. Arachnocides reduce mites.

Pharmacologic: Target therapy to symptoms and on whether symptoms are seasonal or perennial; see **Table 66** and **Table 67**.

Table 66. Choosing Therapy for Allergic Nasal Symptoms				
Agent or Class	**Rhinitis**	**Sneezing**	**Pruritus**	**Congestion**
Glucocorticoids*	+	+	+	+
Ipratropium*	+			
Antihistamines**†	+	+	+	
Pseudoephedrine‡				+
Cromolyn†	+	+	+	+

* Effective in seasonal, perennial, and vasomotor rhinitis.
** Better in seasonal than in perennial rhinitis.
† Start before allergy season.
‡ Topical therapy rapid in onset but results in rebound if used for more than a few days; facilitates use of nasal steroids and sleep during severe attacks.

Table 67. Drug Therapy for Allergic Rhinitis				
Type, Drug	**Geriatric Dosage**	**Formulations**	**Geriatric Half-Life**	**Side Effects**
H₁-Receptor Antagonists or Antihistamines				
√Azelastine (*Astelin*)	2 spr bid**	[topical spr 0.1%, 100 spr]	22–25 h	Bitter taste, nasal burning, sneezing
√Cetirizine (*Zyrtec*)	5 mg/d (max)	[T: 5, 10; syr 5 mg/5mL]	Prolonged	
√Desloratadine (*Clarinex*)	5 mg	[T: 5]	27 h	
Fexofenadine (√*Allegra*, *Allegra-D**)	60 mg po bid; once a day if CrCl < 40; D not recommended	[T: 30, 60, 180; C: 60]	14 h	

(*continues*)

Table 67. Drug Therapy for Allergic Rhinitis (cont.)				
Type, Drug	Geriatric Dosage	Formulations	Geriatric Half-Life	Side Effects
Loratadine (√Claritin, Claritin-D*)	5–10 mg qd; D not recommended	[T: 10; rapid-disintegrating tab 10 mg; syr 1 mg/mL]	Metabolites > 12 d; wide variation	
Chlorpheniramine (eg, Chlor-Trimeton	8–12 mg bid	[T: 4, 8, 12; ChT: 2; CR: 8, 12; S: 2 mg/ 5 mL]	20 h, longer with renal dysfunction	Sedation, dry mouth, confusion, urinary retention; dries lung secretions
Diphenhydramine (eg, Benadryl)	25–50 mg bid	[T: 25, 50; S: elixir 12.5 mg/mL]	13.5 h	Same as chlorpheniramine
Hydroxyzine (eg, Atarax)	25–30 mg bid	[T: 10, 25, 50]	30 h	Same as chlorpheniramine
Decongestants				
Pseudoephedrine (eg, Sudafed, combinations)	60 mg po q 4–6 h	[T: 30, 60; SR: 120; S: elixir 30 mg/5 mL]	2–16 h; varies with urine pH	Arrhythmia, insomnia, anxiety, restlessness, elevated BP
Nasal Steroids				Class side effects: eg,
Beclomethasone (eg, Beconase, Vancenase)	1 spr bid–qid**	[topical spr 16 g (80 spr)]	Rapid absorption, hepatic metabolism	nasal burning, sneezing, bleeding; septal perforation (rare); fungal overgrowth (rare); no significant systemic effects
Budesonide (eg, Rhinocort)	2 spr bid or 4 qd**	[7 g (200 spr)]		
Dexamethasone (eg, Dexacort)	2 spr bid or tid**	[25 mL (200 spr)]		
Flunisolide (eg, Nasalide, Nasarel)	2–4 spr bid or tid**	[25 mL (200 spr)]		
Fluticasone (eg, Flonase)	2 spr qd**	[16 g (120 spr)]		
Mometasone (Nasonex)	2 spr qd**	[17 g (120 spr)]		
Triamcinolone (eg, Nasacort)	2–4 spr qd**	[10 g (100 spr)]		
Other				
Cromolyn (NasalCrom)	1 spr tid–qid;** begin 1–2 wk before exposure to allergen	[2%, 4%]		Nasal irritation, headache, itching of throat

Table 67. Drug Therapy for Allergic Rhinitis (cont.)				
Type, Drug	Geriatric Dosage	Formulations	Geriatric Half-Life	Side Effects
Ipratropium (*Atrovent NS*)	2 spr bid–qid**	[0.03, 0.06%[1] sol]	1.6 h	Epistaxis, nasal irritation, URI, sore throat, nausea. Caution: Do not spray in eyes.

Note: √ = preferred for treating older persons.
* *Allegra-D, Claritin-D* are not recommended; both also contain pseudoephedrine. Contraindicated in narrow angle glaucoma, urinary retention, MAOI use within 14 d, severe hypertension, or CAD. May cause headache, nausea, insomnia.
** Spr per nares.
[†] Use 0.06% for treatment of viral upper respiratory infection.

CHRONIC OBSTRUCTIVE PULMONARY DISEASE

Definition
A spectrum of chronic respiratory diseases characterized by:
- Airflow limitation
- Cough
- Dyspnea
- Frequent pulmonary infection
- Impaired gas exchange
- Sputum production

Therapy
Stepped Approach: Add steps when symptoms inadequately controlled; D/C agent if no improvement. See **Table 68** and **Table 70**.
Smoking Cessation: Essential at any age.
Long-Term Oxygen Therapy: For indications, see **Table 71**.
MDIs: Should be used with an aerochamber; educate patients on use. Use a separate aerochamber for inhaled steroids; wash aerochamber weekly; aerochamber requires separate prescription.

Table 68. COPD Therapy by Severity of Symptoms			
Step	Symptoms	Therapy	Cautions, Comments
1	Mild, intermittent	β_2-Agonist MDI 1–2 puffs q 2–6 h prn	Do not exceed 8–12 puffs/24 h
2	Mild to moderate, continuing	Ipratropium MDI 2–6 puffs q 6–8 h **plus**	Mainstay of therapy
		β_2-Agonist MDI 1–4 puffs qid prn or routine	For rapid relief
3	Suboptimal response or increasing symptoms with step 2 therapy	Add theophylline-SR 200 mg bid **and/or**	Or 400 mg hs for nocturnal bronchospasm
		Albuterol-SR 4–8 mg bid **and/or**	Or at night only
		Mucokinetic agent	If sputum is very viscous

(*continues*)

Table 68. COPD Therapy by Severity of Symptoms (cont.)			
Step	Symptoms	Therapy	Cautions, Comments
4	Persistent symptoms with step 3 therapy	Oral steroids (eg, prednisone) up to 40 mg/d for 10–14 d	With improvement, taper to lowest effective dose, alternate-day dosing, or steroid MDI With no improvement, stop steroid
5	Severe exacerbation	↑ β_2-Agonist, eg, MDI 6–8 puffs q 1/2–2 h or inhalant solution, unit dose every 1/2–2 h, **or** SC epinephrine or terbutaline, 0.1–0.5 mL, **and/or** ↑ Ipratropium MDI 6–8 puffs q 3–4 h **and** Theophylline IV **and** Methylprednisolone IV 50–100 mg STAT and q 6–8 h **and add:** Antibiotic Mucokinetic agent	**Or** inhalant solution 0.5 mg q 4–8 h Calculate to bring serum level to 10–12 μg/mL Taper as soon as possible If indicated If sputum is very viscous

Source: Data in part from Standards for the diagnosis and care of patients with chronic obstructive pulmonary disease: American Thoracic Society. *Am J Respir Crit Care Med.* 1995;152 (5 Pt 2):S77–S121.

ASTHMA
Definition
Chronic inflammatory disorder of the airways; may be triggered by:
- Air pollution
- Allergens
- Chemicals
- Emotional distress
- Exercise
- Tobacco smoke
- Viruses

Characteristics
Can present at any age, but in old age: **cough** is a common presentation, it is less variable and episodic, presents more fixed obstruction, is more difficult to classify. Symptoms:
- Chest tightness
- Cough
- Reversible and variable PEF
- Shortness of breath
- Wheezing

Therapy
Nonpharmacologic: Avoid triggers; educate patients on disease management, use of MDIs, and peak flow meters (document severity and response to therapy).
Pharmacologic: Stepped approach:
- Based on severity of symptoms.
- When symptoms controlled for 3 months, try stepwise reduction.
- If control not achieved, step up, but first review medication technique, adherence, and avoidance of triggers. (See **Table 69**, **Table 70**.)

MDIs should be used with an aerochamber, and patients should be educated on their use. Use separate aerochamber for steroids; wash aerochamber weekly; aerochamber requires separate prescription.

Table 69. Asthma Therapy for Elderly Patients

Step 1. Mild, Intermittent Asthma
Symptom severity: Symptoms < 2/wk; night symptoms: ≤ 2/month, asymptomatic between episodes
PEF/FEV$_1$: ≥ 80% predicted; variability < 20%; normal airflow between attacks.*
Quick-relief therapy: Short-acting: inhaled β_2-agonist < 2/wk. Treatment depends on severity of attack. Inhaled β_2-agonist or cromolyn or nedocromil before exposure to trigger.
Long-term prevention: Avoid triggers. Annual influenza vaccine, pneumococcal vaccine q 6–10 yr. If using β_2-agonists daily or > 1 cannister/mo, step up therapy but review technique first.

Step 2. Moderate Asthma
Symptom severity: Symptoms ≥ 2/wk that affect sleep and activity.
PEF/FEV$_1$: > 60% to ≤ 80% predicted; variability 20% to 30%.
Quick-relief therapy: Short-acting: inhaled β_2-agonist as needed but not to exceed 3–4/d.
Long-term prevention: Daily medications: inhaled corticosteroid, 200–2000 μg preferred. Cromolyn, montelukast, nedocromil have not been studied in older people. Theophylline-SR has many interactions and side effects. If needed, add long-acting inhaled β_2-agonist. If there is fixed obstruction, add ipratropium.

Step 3. Severe, Persistent Asthma
Symptom severity: Continuous symptoms, limited physical activity, frequent night symptoms.
PEF/FEV$_1$: ≤ 60% predicted; variability > 30%.
Quick-relief therapy: Short-acting: inhaled β_2-agonist as needed for symptoms, not to exceed 3–4/d.
Long-term prevention: Daily medications: inhaled corticosteroid, 800–2000 μg or more, and either long-acting inhaled β_2-agonist or theophylline-SR and/or ipratropium, and oral corticosteroid.

Step 4. Severe Exacerbations
Symptom severity: Difficulty speaking sentences, walking; fingernails or lips turned blue.
Quick-relief therapy: Evaluation: ABG, ECG, CXR, serum K$^+$. Treat with aerosolized β_2-agonist q 20–30 min × 1 h with continuous ECG monitoring. Nasal O$_2$ to keep sats > 92%. Avoid theophylline for the first 4 h. Antibiotics for change in sputum. Avoid overhydration.

* Some degree of fixed obstruction is common in older asthmatics. To determine irreversibility, FEV$_1$ or PEF before and after prednisone. 0.3–1 mg/kg/d × 2 wk.
Source: Adapted from National Asthma Education and Prevention Program, *NAEPP Working Group Report: Considerations for Diagnosing and Managing Asthma in the Elderly.* Bethesda, MD: National Heart, Lung, and Blood Institute; Feb. 1996. NIH Publication No. 96-3662.

Table 70. Asthma and COPD Medications

Drug	Dosage	Side Effects (Metabolism, Excretion)
Anticholinergics		
√ Ipratropium (*Atrovent*)	2–6 puffs qid or 0.5 mg by nebulizer qid	Dry mouth, bitter taste (Lung; poorly absorbed)
Short-acting β_2-Agonists*		Class side effects include tremor, nervousness, headache, palpitations, tachycardia, cough, hypokalemia. Caution: use half-doses in persons with known or suspected coronary disease (L)
√ Albuterol (*Proventil, Ventolin*)	2–6 puffs q 4–6 h or 2.5 mg by nebulizer qid; 1.5–3.5 mg bid–qid by nebulizer; ER tablets 4–8 mg po q 12 h	

(continues)

Table 70. Asthma and COPD Medications (cont.)		
Drug	**Dosage**	**Side Effects (Metabolism, Excretion)**
Albuterol (*Ventolin Rotacaps*)	1–2 caps q 4–6 h; dry powder inhaler 200 μg/inhalation	
√ Bitolterol (*Tornalate*)	1–3 puffs q 4–6 h	
Isoetharine (eg, *Bronkometer, Bronkosol*)	0.25–0.5 mL of 1% sol; 2 mL NS by nebulizer q 1–4 h; inhaler 1–2 puffs q 4 h	Use limited by short duration of action; not widely used for this reason
Levalbuterol (*Xopenex*)	0.63 mg q 6–8 h	Expensive; no advantage over racemic albuterol
Pirbuterol (*Maxair*)	2–3 puffs q 4–6 h	Mechanism may be difficult for older patients to trigger
Long-acting β-Agonists		Class side effects include tremor, nervousness, headache, palpitations, tachycardia, cough, hypokalemia; caution: use half-doses in persons with known or suspected coronary disease; not for acute exacerbation (L)
√ Salmeterol (*Serevent*)	2 puffs bid	
√ Formoterol (*Foradil*)	1 puff q 12 h	Onset of action 1–3 min
Corticosteroids: Inhaled		Class side effects include nausea, vomiting, diarrhea, abdominal pain; oropharyngeal thrush; dosages > 1.0 mg/d may cause adrenal suppression, reduce calcium absorption and bone density, and cause bruising (L)
√ Beclomethasone (*Beclovent, Vanceril*)	2–4 puffs bid–qid [42, 84 μg/puff, max 840 mg/d]	
√ Budesonide (eg, *Pulmicort*)	1–2 puffs bid–qid [100, 200, 400 μg/puff]	
√ Dexamethasone (eg, *Dexacort*)	3 puffs tid–qid [100 μg/puff]	
√ Flunisolide (eg, *AeroBid*)	2–4 puffs bid [250 μg/puff]	
√ Fluticasone (eg, *Flovent*)	1 puff bid [44, 110, 220 μg/puff]	
√ Triamcinolone (eg, *Azmacort*)	2 puffs tid–qid or 4 puffs bid [100 μg/puff]	
Corticosteroids: Oral		
Prednisone (eg, *Deltasone, Orasone*)	20 mg po bid [T: 1, 2.5, 5, 10, 20, 50; elixir 5 mg/5 mL]	Leukocytosis, thrombocytosis, sodium retention, euphoria, depression, hallucination, cognitive dysfunction; other effects with long-term use (L)
Long-acting Theophyllines		Class side effects include atrial arrhythmias, seizures, increased gastric acid secretion, ulcer, reflux, diuresis (L**)
(eg, *Quibron-T/SR*)	300–400 mg/d [T: 300 bisect, trisect tabs]	
(eg, *Theo-Dur, Slo-Bid*)	100–200 mg po bid [T: 100, 200, 300, 450]	
(eg, *Uniphyl, Theo-24*)	400 mg po qd [T: 100, 200, 300, 400]	

Table 70. Asthma and COPD Medications (cont.)		
Drug	Dosage	Side Effects (Metabolism, Excretion)
Leukotriene Modifiers		
Montelukast (*Singulair*)	10 mg po in AM [T: 10; ChT: 4, 5]	Unknown, minimal data in elderly patients; leukotriene-receptor antagonist (L)
Zafirlukast (*Accolate*)	20 mg po bid 1 h before or 2 h after meals [T: 10, 20]	Headache, somnolence, dizziness, nausea, diarrhea, abdominal pain, fever; monitor LFTs; monitor coumarin anticoagulants; leukotriene-receptor antagonist (L, reduced by 50% > 65 yr)
Zileuton (*Zyflo*)	600 mg po qid [T: 600]	Dizziness, insomnia, nausea, abdominal pain, abnormal LFTs, myalgia; monitor coumarin anticoagulants; other drug interactions; inhibits synthesis of leukotrienes (L)
Other Medications		
√ Albuterol-Ipratropium (*Combivent*)	0.09/0.018 mg/puff, 2–3 puffs qid; 3 mg/ 0.5 mg by nebulizer qid	Same as individual agents (L, K)
Cromolyn sodium (eg, *Intal*)	2–4 puffs or 20-mg caps qid	Because of propellant, use MDI with caution in coronary disease or arrhythmia (L, K)
Nedocromil (*Tilade*)	2 puffs qid	Bitter taste, headache, dizziness, sore throat, cough, chest tightness (K, F)
Salmeterol-Fluticasone combination (*Advair Diskus*)	1 puff bid (50 μg/100, 250, or 500 μg/ inhalation)	

Note: √ = preferred for treating older persons.
* Older nonselective β_2-agonists such as isoproterenol, metoproterenol, epinephrine are not recommended and are more toxic.
** Clearance reduced by 30% in older patients. Caution: Initial dosage for older patients should not exceed 400 mg/d. Follow blood levels to adjust up or down for individual patients.

Table 71. Indications for Long-Term Oxygen Therapy			
Pao$_2$ Level	Sao$_2$ Level	Other	Need
$\leq$ 55 mm Hg	$\leq$ 88%	–	Absolute
55–59 mm Hg	$\geq$ 89%	Signs of tissue hypoxia (ie, cor pulmonale by ECG, CHF, hematocrit > 55%)	Yes
$\geq$ 60 mm Hg	$\geq$ 90%	Desaturation with exercise	Yes*
		Desaturation with sleep apnea not corrected by CPAP	Yes*

* If patient meets criteria at rest, oxygen should also be prescribed during sleep and exercise, appropriately titrated. If patient is normoexemic at rest but desaturates during exercise or sleep (Pao$_2$ $\leq$ 55 mm Hg), oxygen should be prescribed. Also consider CPAP or BIPAP.
Source: Data from Standards for the diagnosis and care of patients with chronic obstructive pulmonary disease: American Thoracic Society. *Am J Respir Crit Care Med.* 1995;152 (5 Pl 2):S77–S121.

COUGH

Cough is a symptom of many acute and chronic respiratory and cardiac illnesses. Therapy first identifies, then treats the underlying problem. Chronic rhinitis is the most common cause of cough in older people (see **Table 67**). For symptomatic relief of cough, the agents in **Table 72** may be helpful.

Table 72. Antitussives and Expectorants			
Drug	Dosage	Formulations	Comments (Metabolism)
Benzonatate* (*Tessalon Perles*)	100 mg po tid (max: 600 mg/d)	[C: 100, 200]	Side effects: CNS stimulation or depression, headache, dizziness, hallucination, constipation (L)
Dextromethorphan** (eg, *Robitussin DM*)	10–30 mL po q 4–8 h	[C: 30; S: 10 mg/ 5 mL]	Side effects: mild drowsiness, fatigue; interacts with fluoxetine, paroxetine; combination may cause serotonin syndrome (L)
Guaifenesin** (eg, *Robitussin*)	5–20 mL po q 4 h	[S: 100 mg/5 mL]	Side effects: none at low doses; high doses cause nausea, vomiting, diarrhea, drowsiness, abdominal pain (L)
*Histussin HC***	10 mL q 4 h up to 40 mL/d	[S: hydrocodone 2.5 mg + phenylephrine 5 mg + chlor-pheniramine 2 mg/mL]	Side effects: sedation, constipation, nervousness, tachycardia, hypertension, urinary retention (L)
Hydrocodone** (*Hycodan*)	5 mL po q 4–6 h	[S: 5 mg/5 mL]	Side effects include sedation, constipation, confusion (L)

Note: * = antitussive and expectorant; ** = antitussive.

PULMONARY EMBOLISM

Symptoms

Classic triad—dyspnea, chest pain, hemoptysis—occurs in ≤ 20% of cases. Consider PE with any of the following:

- Chest pain
- Hypotension
- Shortness of breath
- Tachycardia
- Hemoptysis
- Hypoxia
- Syncope

Diagnosis

- Ventilation-perfusion (V-P) lung scans: normal scan reduces probability of PE to 4% in a high-risk setting and effectively excludes PE in an average or low-probability setting; a high-probability scan has a sensitivity of 41% and positive predictive value of 87% in high-risk settings. With low risk of complications and a high-probability scan, begin

treatment for PE; intermediate or low-probability scans are nondiagnostic and are not sufficient to exclude PE.
- D-dimer $< 500\ \mu$g/L excludes PE with a nondiagnostic V-P$_R$ scan.
- Ultrasound of the lower limbs positive for DVT warrants anticoagulation without other testing.
- Spiral-chest CT has not received adequate evaluation as a noninvasive diagnostic for PE.
- Pulmonary angiography is most accurate, false negative is 0% to 10%; complication rate 5%; mortality 1–4/1000.

Pharmacologic Therapy
- Standard therapy for PE remains IV heparin followed by warfarin.
  - Heparin (see **Table 11**): mix infusion 100 units/mL in D5W; cleared through the reticuloendothelial system, half-life of anticoagulation effect 1.5 h
  - Warfarin (see p 17 and **Table 9**)
- Low-molecular-weight heparins (LMWH) appear safe and effective for both DVT and PE.
  - LMWH (see **Table 12**)
- Acute massive PE (filling defects in 2 or more lobar arteries, or the equivalent, by angiogram) associated with hypotension or severe hypoxia or high pulmonary pressures on ECG should usually be treated with thrombolytic therapy within 48 h of onset. (See **Table 12**)

SEXUAL DYSFUNCTION

IMPOTENCE (ERECTILE DYSFUNCTION)

Definition
Inability to achieve erection sufficient for intercourse. Prevalence nearly 70% by age 70.

Causes
Often multifactorial; > 50% of cases arterial, venous, or mixed vascular cause. Also:

- Diabetes mellitus
- Drug side effects
- Hyperprolactinemia
- Hypogonadism
- Neurologic: eg, disorders of the CNS, spinal cord, or PNS; autonomic neuropathy; temporal lobe epilepsy
- Psychologic: eg, depression, anxiety, bereavement
- Thyroid or adrenal disorders

Decreased bioavailable testosterone is more associated with decreased libido than with erectile dysfunction.

Evaluation
History: Type and duration of problem; relation to surgery, trauma, medication. Problems with orgasm, libido, or penile detumescence are not erectile dysfunction.

Physical Findings:
- Neuropathy: orthostatic hypotension, impaired response to Valsalva's maneuver, absent bulbocavernosus or cremasteric reflexes
- Peyronie's disease: penile bands, plaques
- Hypogonadism: diminished male pattern hair, gynecomastia, small (< 20–25 mm long) testes

Assessment:
- Reduced penile-to-brachial pressure index suggests vascular disease.
- Cavernosometry diagnoses venous leak syndrome; reserved for surgical candidates.
- Test dose of prostaglandin E or papaverine can exclude vascular disease or confirm venous leak syndrome.
- For libido problems check total and bioavailable testosterone, luteinizing hormone, TSH, and prolactin.

Therapy

Table 73. Management of Erectile Dysfunction		
Cause	**Therapy**	**Comments**
Hypogonadism, poor libido	Testosterone: scrotal transdermal (*Testoderm*) [4, 5, 6] 4–6 mg qd; *or* skin transdermal (*Androderm*) [2.5, 5] 5 mg/d; *or* testosterone cypionate or enanthate 200 mg IM q 2–4 wk	When given IM, can cause polycythemia, potential for increased prostate size, fluid retention, gynecomastia, liver dysfunction, but IM testosterone is inexpensive and generally well tolerated

Table 73. Management of Erectile Dysfunction (cont.)		
Cause	Therapy	Comments
	or testosterone gel 1% (*AndroGel*) [5 g (50 mg/24 h), 7.5 g (75 mg), 10 g (100 mg)] begin with 5 g pk qam	Squeeze pk contents into palm of hand and apply, let dry; wash hands immediately. Check serum testosterone after 14 d and adjust dose; do not use in women.
Neuropathic, vascular, or mixed	Vacuum tumescence devices (*Osbon-Erec Aid, Catalyst Vacuum Device, Pos-T-Vac, Rejoyn*)	Rare: Ecchymosis, reduced ejaculation, coolness of penile tip. Good acceptance in older population; intercourse successful in 70% to 90% of cases
	Intracavernosal [5, 10, 20, 40 μg] *or* intraurethral [125, 250, 500, 1000 μg] prostaglandin E (*Alprostadil*)	Risks: hypotension, bruising, bleeding, priapism; erection > 4 h requires emergency treatment; intraurethral safer and more acceptable
	Penile prosthesis	Complications: infection, mechanical failure, penile fibrosis
Organic, psychogenic, or mixed	Sildenafil (*Viagra*) [25, 50, 100] start 25 mg 1 h before sexual activity; maximum 1/d	Contraindicated with use of nitrates; caution in vascular disease; least effective in vascular impotence. Several other drug interactions; metabolism reduced in liver and kidney disease, and aging. Side effects: headache, flushing, dyspepsia (mild and transient), color tinge in vision, nasal congestion, UTI, diarrhea, dizziness, and rash

DYSPAREUNIA
Definition
Pain with intercourse.

Aggravating Factors
- Gynecologic tumors
- Interstitial cystitis
- Myalgia from overexertion during Kegel's exercises
- Osteoarthritis
- Pelvic fractures
- Retroverted uterus
- Sacral nerve root compression
- Vaginal atrophy from estrogen deprivation
- Vulvar or vaginal infection

Evaluation
- Ask about sexual problems (eg, changes in libido, partner's function, and health issues).
- Screen for depression.
- Perform pelvic examination for vulvovaginitis, vaginal atrophy, conization (decreased distensibility and narrowing of the vaginal canal), scarring, pelvic inflammatory disease, cystocele, and rectocele.

Management
- Identify and treat clinical pathology.
- Educate and counsel patients.
- Discuss hormone replacement therapy (see pp 167–169).
- Water-soluble lubricants (eg, *Replens*) are highly effective as monotherapy for those who cannot or will not use hormones, or as a supplement to estrogen.
- For vaginismus (vaginal muscle spasm), trial cessation of intercourse and gradual vaginal dilation may help.
- For diminished libido, short-term use of androgens (which used long-term adversely affect health) may help; refer for counseling or sex therapy.
- For atrophic vaginitis: estrogen cream, use minimum dose (eg, 0.5 g *Premarin* [42.5 g], 2 g *Ogen* or *Estrace* [42.5 g]), daily for 2 wk, then 1–3 × /wk thereafter; estradiol vaginal ring (*Estring*) inserted intravaginally and changed q 90 d, high degree of safety and acceptability; estradiol vaginal tablets (*Vagifem* 25 μg) inserted intravaginally daily × 2 wk, then twice/wk.

SSRI-INDUCED SEXUAL DYSFUNCTION
- Incidence varies widely, from 1% to 20% of patients making spontaneous reports to 75% when patients are systematically questioned.
- Symptoms include anorgasmia, decreased libido, and ejaculatory dysfunction.
- Tolerance may develop up to 12 wk on treatment.
- Pharmacologic management:
  - For sertraline and citalopram (not other SSRIs), reducing dose or drug holidays (skip or reduce weekend dose) may help.
  - Adjuvant medications reported as effective for this condition in case reports include
    - Bupropion (*Wellbutrin SR, Zyban*) 75–100 mg po qd
    - Mirtazapine (*Remeron*) 15 mg po hs
    - Sildenafil (*Viagra*) 25–100 mg 1 h before intercourse

SLEEP DISORDERS

CLASSIFICATION
- Disturbance of the sleep-wake cycle
- Hypersomnolence
- Insomnia (difficulty initiating or maintaining sleep)
- Parasomnias (disorders of arousal, partial arousal, and sleep stage transition)
- Sleep apnea

SLEEP DISORDERS OTHER THAN SLEEP APNEA
Risk Factors and Aggravating Factors
Treatable Associated Medical and Psychiatric Conditions: Adjustment disorders, anxiety, bereavement, cough, depression, dyspnea (cardiac or pulmonary), GERD, nocturia, pain, paresthesias, stress
Medications That Cause or Aggravate Sleep Problems: Alcohol, antidepressants, β-blockers, bronchodilators, caffeine, clonidine, cortisone, diuretics, levodopa, methyldopa, nicotine, phenytoin, progesterone, quinidine, reserpine, sedatives, sympathomimetics including decongestants

Management
Sleep improvements are better sustained over time with behavioral treatment.
Nonpharmacologic—Measures Recommended to Improve Sleep Hygiene:
- During the daytime:
  - Get out of bed at the same time each morning regardless of how much you slept the night before.
  - Exercise daily, but not immediately before bedtime.
  - Get adequate exposure to bright light during the day.
  - Decrease or eliminate naps, unless necessary part of sleeping schedule.
  - Limit or eliminate alcohol, caffeine, and nicotine, especially before bedtime.
- At bedtime:
  - Maintain a regular sleeping time, but don't go to bed unless sleepy.
  - If hungry, have a light snack before bed (unless there are symptoms of GERD or it is otherwise medically contraindicated), but avoid heavy meals at bedtime.
  - Don't read or watch television in bed.
  - Relax mentally before going to sleep; don't use bedtime as worry time.
  - Relax before bedtime, and maintain a routine period of preparation for bed (eg, washing up and going to the bathroom).
  - Control the nighttime environment with comfortable temperature, quietness, darkness.
  - Wear comfortable bedclothes.
  - If it helps, use soothing noise, for example, a fan or other appliance or a "white noise" machine.
  - If unable to fall asleep within 15–20 min, get out of bed and perform soothing activity, such as listening to soft music or reading (but avoid exposure to bright light during these times).

Pharmacologic—Principles of Prescribing Medications for Sleep Disorders:
- Use lowest effective dose.
- Use intermittent dosing (2–4 times/wk).
- Prescribe medications for short-term use (no more than 3–4 wk).
- Discontinue medication gradually.
- Be alert for rebound insomnia following discontinuation.

Table 74 Useful Medications for Sleep Disorders in Elderly Persons				
Class, Drug	**Usual Dose**	**Formulations**	**Half-Life**	**Comments (Metabolism, Excretion)**
Antidepressant, sedating				
Nefazodone (*Serzone*)	50–200 mg	[T: 50, 100, 150, 200, 250]	2–4 h	Antianxiety effect; less orthostasis than with trazodone; hepatotoxicity, obtain baseline LFT (L)
Trazodone (*Desyrel*)	25–150 mg	[T: 50, 100, 150, 300]	12 h	Moderate orthostatic effects; effective for insomnia with or without depression (L)
Benzodiazepine, intermediate-acting				
Estazolam (*ProSom*)	0.5–1.0 mg	[T: 1, 2]	12–18 h	Rapidly absorbed, effective in initiating sleep; slightly active metabolites that may accumulate (K)
Lorazepam (*Ativan*)	0.25–2 mg	[T: 0.5, 1, 2]	8–12 h	Effective in initiating and maintaining sleep; associated with falls, memory loss, rebound insomnia (K)
Temazepam (*Restoril*)	7.5–15 mg	[C: 7.5, 15, 30]	8–10 h*	Daytime drowsiness may occur with repeated use; effective for sleep maintenance; delayed onset of effect (K)
Nonbenzodiazepine, short-acting				
Zaleplon (*Sonata*)	5 mg	[C: 5, 10]	1 h	Avoid taking with alcohol or food (L)
Zolpidem (*Ambien*)	5 mg	[T: 5, 10]	1.5–4.5 h**	Confusion and agitation may occur but are rare (L)
CNS depressant, nonbarbiturate and nonbenzodiazepine				
Chloral hydrate (*Aquachloral, Supprettes*)	500–1000 mg (not to exceed 2 g as single dose or total daily dose)	[C: 500; syr 500 mg/ 5 mL; Sp: 324, 500, 648]	8 h (active metabolite)	Hypnotic effect lost after 2 wk of continuous use; contraindicated in marked cardiac, hepatic, or renal impairment (K, L)
Hormone				
Melatonin	0.3–5 mg	[various]	1 h	Not regulated by FDA

* Can be as long as 30 h in elderly persons.
** 3 h in elderly persons; 10 h in those with hepatic cirrhosis.

SLEEP APNEA

Definition

Repeated episodes of apnea (cessation of airflow for ≥ 10 sec) or hypopnea (transient reduction [$\geq 30\%$ decrease in thoracoabdominal movement or airflow and with at least 4% oxygen desaturation or an arousal] of airflow for ≥ 10 sec) during sleep with excessive daytime sleepiness or altered cardiopulmonary function.

Classification

Obstructive (90% of cases): Airflow cessation as a result of upper airway closure in spite of adequate respiratory muscle effort
Central: Cessation of respiratory effort
Mixed: Features of both obstructive and central

Associated Risk Factors, Clinical Features

Family hx, HTN, increased neck circumference, male gender, obesity, smoking, snoring, upper airway structural abnormalities (eg, soft palate, tonsils)

Evaluation

- Full night's sleep study (polysomnography) in sleep laboratory indicated for those who habitually snore and either report daytime sleepiness or have observed apnea.
- Results are reported as the apnea-hypopnea index (AHI), which is the number of episodes of apneas and hypopneas per hour of sleep.
- Threshold for CPAP reimbursement by Medicare based on a minimum of 2 h sleep by polysomnography is AHI (1) ≥ 15 or (2) ≥ 5 and ≤ 14 with documented symptoms of excessive daytime sleepiness, impaired cognition, mood disorders, or insomnia, or documented HTN, ischemic heart disease, or hx of stroke.

Management

Nonpharmacologic:

- Use CPAP by nasal mask, nasal prongs, or mask that covers the nose and mouth (considered initial treatment for clinically important sleep apnea).
- Avoid use of alcohol or sedatives.
- Lie in lateral rather than supine position; may be facilitated by soft foam ball in a backpack.
- Lose weight (obese patients).
- Use oral appliances that keep the tongue in an anterior position during sleep or keep the mandible forward.

Pharmacologic: Beneficial mostly in mild sleep apnea.

- Protriptyline (*Vivactil*) 10–20 mg/d [T: 5, 10] L (men commonly experience urinary hesitancy or frequency and impotence)
- Fluoxetine (*Prozac*) 10–20 mg [T: 10, 20, 40; S: 20 mg/5 mL] L

Surgical:

- Tracheostomy (indicated for patients with severe apnea who cannot tolerate positive pressure or when other interventions are ineffective)
- Uvulopalatopharyngoplasty (curative in fewer than 50% of cases)
- Maxillofacial surgery (rare cases)

OTHER CONDITIONS ASSOCIATED WITH SLEEP DISORDERS
Nocturnal Leg Cramps
Stretching exercises may be helpful. Quinine, 200–300 mg po hs [T: 200, 260, 300, 325] may reduce the frequency though not the severity of leg cramps. Cinchonism, hemolysis, thrombocytopenia, and visual disturbances are notable side effects.

Restless Legs Syndrome
Diagnostic Criteria:
- Vague discomfort, usually bilateral, most commonly in calves
- Symptoms exacerbated by rest, especially at night
- Symptoms relieved by movement—jerking, stretching, or shaking of limbs; pacing

Nonpharmacologic Treatment:
- Exclude or treat iron deficiency, peripheral neuropathy.
- Avoid alcohol, caffeine, nicotine.
- If possible, avoid SSRIs, TCAs, lithium, and dopamine antagonists.
- Rub limbs.
- Use hot or cold baths, whirlpools.

Pharmacologic Treatment: Start at low dose, increase as needed:
- First line: carbidopa-levodopa (*Sinemet*) 25/100 mg, 1–2 h prior to bedtime. Patients may develop symptom augmentation that occurs earlier in the day (eg, afternoon instead of evening) and may be more severe. Treatment of augmentation may require reduction of dose or switch to dopamine agonist.
- Second-line agents include dopamine agonists (see **Table 53**), carbamazepine (see **Table 54**), and gabapentin (see **Table 54**).
- For refractory cases, benzodiazepines or opioids can be tried.

Periodic Limb Movement Disorder
Diagnostic Criteria:
- Insomnia or excessive sleepiness
- Repetitive, highly stereotyped limb muscle movements (eg, extension of big toes with partial flexion of ankle, knee, and sometimes hip)
- Polysomnographic monitoring showing repetitive episodes of muscle contractions and associated arousals or awakenings
- No evidence of a medical, mental, or other sleep disorder that can account for symptoms

Treatment: Indicated for clinically significant sleep disruption or frequent arousals documented on a sleep study.
- Nonpharmacologic: cognitive-behavioral therapy
- Pharmacologic: See restless legs syndrome, above.

URINARY INCONTINENCE

DEFINITION
UI is not a normal part of aging. It is a loss of urine control due to a combination of
- Genitourinary pathology
- Age-related changes
- Comorbid conditions
- Environmental obstacles

CLASSIFICATION
Reversible Causes of Incontinence (DRIP Mnemonic)
Delirium
Restricted mobility (illness, injury, gait disorder, restraint)
Infection (acute, symptomatic); **I**nflammation (atrophic vaginitis); **I**mpaction of stool
Polyuria (diabetes mellitus, caffeine intake, volume overload); **P**harmaceuticals
(diuretics, autonomic agents, psychotropics)

Established Incontinence
Urge: Detrusor muscle overactivity (uninhibited bladder contractions); small to large
volume loss; may be idiopathic or associated with CNS lesions or bladder irritation from
infection, stones, tumors; may be associated with impaired contractility and retention
(detrusor hyperactivity with impaired contractility, or DHIC).
Stress: Failure of sphincter mechanisms to remain closed during bladder filling (often
due to insufficient pelvic support in women and trauma from prostate surgery in men);
loss occurs with increased intra-abdominal pressure.
Overflow: Impaired detrusor contractility or bladder outlet obstruction. Impaired
contractility—chronic outlet obstruction, diabetes mellitus, vitamin B_{12} deficiency,
tabes dorsalis, alcoholism, or spinal disease. Outlet obstruction—in men, BPH, cancer,
stricture; in women, prior incontinence surgery or large cystocele.
Mixed: Combined urge and stress UI is common in older women.
Functional: Inability or unwillingness to toilet because of physical, cognitive,
psychologic, or environmental factors.
Other (Rare): Bladder-sphincter dyssynergia, fistulas, reduced detrusor compliance,
recurrent cystitis.

RISK FACTORS
- Age-related changes (BPH, atrophic urethritis)
- CHF, nocturia, COPD, or chronic cough
- Constipation
- Dementia, depression, stroke, Parkinson's disease
- Detrusor overactivity and uninhibited contractions
- Fecal incontinence
- Increased postvoid residual or decreased bladder capacity
- Impaired ADLs
- Obesity

EVALUATION

History
- Precipitant urgency suggests detrusor overactivity.
- Loss with cough, laugh, or bend suggests stress.
- Continuous leakage suggests intrinsic sphincter insufficiency or overflow.
- Onset, frequency, volume, timing, precipitants (eg, caffeine, diuretics, alcohol, cough, medications).

Physical Examination
- Functional status (eg, mobility, dexterity)
- Mental status
- Orthostatic BP, HR
- Findings:
  - Bladder distension
  - Cervical cord compression (interosseus muscle wasting, Hoffmann's or Babinski's signs)
  - Rectal mass or impaction
  - Sacral root integrity (anal sphincter tone, anal wink, perineal sensation)
  - Volume overload, edema

Male GU
Prostate consistency; symmetry; for uncircumcised, check phimosis, paraphimosis, balanitis

Female GU
Atrophic vaginitis; pelvic support (see also pp 154, 168)

Testing
Voiding Record: Record time and volume of incontinent, continent episodes; activities and time of sleep; knowing oral intake is sometimes helpful.
Standing Full Bladder Stress Test: Relax perineum and cough once—immediate loss suggests stress, several seconds' delay suggests detrusor overactivity.
Postvoid Residual: If > 100 mL, repeat; still > 100 mL suggests detrusor weakness, neuropathy, outlet obstruction, or DHIC.
Laboratory: UA and urine C&S; glucose and calcium if polyuric; renal function tests and B_{12} if urinary retention; urine cytology if hematuria or pain; PSA if cancer suspected.
Urodynamic Testing: Not routinely indicated; indicated before corrective surgery, when diagnosis is unclear, or when empiric therapy fails.

MANAGEMENT
In a stepped approach, treat all transient causes first (DRIP); avoid caffeine, alcohol, minimize evening intake of fluids.

Nonpharmacologic Behavioral Therapy (First-Line Therapy)
Detrusor Instability: Timed toileting—shortest interval to keep dry; urge control—when urgency occurs, sit or stand quietly, focus on letting urge pass, when no longer urgent

walk slowly to the bathroom and void. When no incontinence for 2 d, increase voiding interval by 30–60 min until voiding every 3–4 h. Electrical stimulation often effective; refer to PT. Pelvic muscle exercises (see below).

Cognitively Impaired Persons: Prompted toileting (ask if patient needs to void) at 2- to 3-h intervals during day; encourage patients to report continence status; praise patient when continent and responds to toileting.

Stress Incontinence: Pelvic muscle (Kegel's) exercises—isolate pelvic muscles (avoid thigh, rectal, buttocks contraction); perform 3–10 sets of 10 contractions at maximum strength daily; progressively longer (up to 10-sec) contractions; follow-up and encouragement necessary; consider biofeedback for training or have patient practice interrupting urine stream while voiding.

Pessaries: May benefit women with vaginal or uterine prolapse.

DHIC: Treat urge first; self-intermittent clean catheterization if needed.

Pharmacologic Therapy

Estrogen replacement may benefit both urge and stress UI in patients with atrophic urethritis; see **Table 78** for recommended dose regimens. Topical estrogens are also effective; see p 154 for available preparations. See **Table 75** for other therapies.

Table 75. Drugs to Treat Urinary Incontinence, by Types			
R_x by UI Type	Dosage	Formulations	Comments (Metabolism)
Urge or Mixed UI*			
Dicyclomine (*Bentyl*)	10–20 mg tid	[T: 20; C: 10; S: syr 10 mg/5 mL]	Dry mouth, blurry vision, ↑ intraocular pressure, delirium, constipation, plus postural ↓ BP, cardiac conduction disturbances (K)
Hyoscyamine (*Anaspaz, Cystospaz, Levsin*)	0.375–0.75 mg qid 0.375–0.75 po q 12 h	[T: 0.125; S: elixir 0.125 mg/5 mL] [SR: 0.375]	May exhibit less dry mouth, depending on dosage; delirium, nervousness, insomnia (K)
Imipramine (*Tofranil*)	10–50 mg qd	[T: 10, 25, 50]	Dry mouth, blurry vision, ↑ intraocular pressure, delirium, constipation, plus postural ↓ BP, cardiac conduction disturbances (L)
✓ Oxybutynin (*Ditropan, Ditropan XL*)	2.5–5.0 mg bid–tid 5–20 mg qd	[T: 5; S: 5 mg/ 5 mL] [SR: 5, 10, 15]	Dry mouth, blurry vision, ↑ intraocular pressure, delirium, constipation (L)
Propantheline (*Pro-Banthine*)	15–30 mg tid (on empty stomach)	[T: 15]	Dry mouth, blurry vision, ↑ intraocular pressure, delirium, constipation (L, K)
Flavoxate (*Urispas*)	100–200 mg tid–qid	[T: 100]	Tachycardia, palpitations, drowsiness, delirium, nausea, vomiting, dry mouth, ↑ intraocular pressure (L, K)
✓ Tolterodine (*Detrol, Detrol LA*)	2 mg bid 4 mg qd	[T: 1, 2] [C: ER 2, 4]	Dry mouth, dyspepsia, constipation, delirium (L)

(continues)

Table 75. Drugs to Treat Urinary Incontinence, by Types (cont.)			
Rx by UI Type	Dosage	Formulations	Comments (Metabolism)
Stress UI†			
Pseudoephedrine (eg, *Sudafed*)	15–30 mg tid	[T: 30, 60; elixir 30 mg/5 mL]	Headache, tachycardia, ↑ BP (L)
(*Sudafed XR*)	120 mg qd, bid	[SR: 120]	

Note: √ = preferred in treating older people. For prostate obstruction UI, see p 141.
* Drugs to treat urge or mixed UI: ↑ bladder capacity, ↓ involuntary contractions.
† Drugs to treat stress UI: ↑ urethral smooth muscle contraction.

Surgical Therapy

Patients with stress incontinence or intrinsic sphincter deficiency who do not respond to behavioral or pharmacologic therapy should be considered for surgery. Evaluation should include complete urodynamic studies. Case-control studies indicate a cure rate of 59% to 92%, with an additional 4% to 25% improved. Complication rates vary from 6% for bulking techniques to 32% for artificial sphincters.

CATHETER CARE

- Use **only** for chronic urinary retention, nonhealing pressure ulcers in incontinent patients, and when requested by patients or families to promote comfort.
- Use closed drainage system only; avoid topical or systemic antibiotics or catheters treated with antibiotics. Silver alloy hydrogel catheters reduce UTI by 27% to 73%.
- Bacteriuria is universal; treat only if symptoms (ie, fever, inanition, anorexia, delirium), or if bacteriuria persists after catheter removal.
- How to culture from catheter: through the port, not from the bag.
- Replace catheter if symptomatic bacteriuria occurs, then culture urine.
- Nursing facility patients with catheters should be kept in separate rooms.
- For acute retention catheterize for 7–10 d, then do voiding trial after catheter removal, never clamping.
- **Replacing Catheters:** Routine replacement not necessary. Changing every 4–6 wk is reasonable to prevent blockage. Patients with recurrent blockage need increased fluid intake and dilute acetic acid bladder irrigation.

VISUAL IMPAIRMENT

DEFINITION
Visual acuity 20/40 or worse; severe visual impairment (legal blindness) 20/200 or worse

EVALUATION
Acuity Testing
Near Vision: Check each eye independently with glasses using handheld Rosenbaum card at 14" or Lighthouse Near Acuity Test at 16".
Far Vision: Snellen wall chart at 20'
Visual Fields: By confrontation

Ophthalmoscopic Evaluation

Tonometry using Tono-pen (portable)

Causes of Visual Impairment in Decreasing Order of Frequency
Refractive Error: Most common cause of impairment
Cataracts: Lens opacity on ophthalmoscopic examination. Risk factors: Age, sun exposure, smoking, corticosteroids, diabetes mellitus.
Age-Related Macular Degeneration (ARMD): Atrophy of cells in the central macular region of retinal pigmented epithelium; on ophthalmoscopic examination white-yellow patches (drusen) or hemorrhage and scars in advanced stages. Risk factors: Age, sunlight exposure, family hx, white race.
Diabetic Retinopathy: Microaneurysms, dot and blot hemorrhages on ophthalmoscopy with proliferative retinopathy ischemia and vitreous hemorrhage. Risk factors: Chronic hyperglycemia.
Glaucoma: Intraocular pressure > 21 mm Hg, optic cupping and nerve head atrophy, and loss of peripheral visual fields. Risk factors: Black race, age, family hx, elevated eye pressures.

MANAGEMENT
Prevention:
Biennial full eye examinations for persons > 65 years of age, annually for diabetic persons

Nonpharmacologic Interventions
ARMD: Photocoagulation for wet form: monitor using Amsler grid daily.
Cataract Surgery: AHCPR guidelines (AHCPR Publication No. 93-0542): if acuity 20/50 or worse with symptoms of poor functional acuity; or if 20/40 or better with disabling glare or frequent exposure to low light situations, diplopia, disparity between eyes, or occupational need; or when cataract removal will treat another lens-induced disease (eg, glaucoma); or when cataract coexists with retinal disease requiring unrestricted monitoring (eg, diabetic retinopathy)
Diabetic Retinopathy: Laser treatment of proliferative retinopathy or macular edema

Glaucoma Surgery: Open angle—laser trabeculoplasty or surgical trabeculectomy; angle closure—laser iridotomy; used primarily when pressures are poorly controlled by topical agents or when visual loss progresses

Pharmacologic Interventions

ARMD: Zinc oxide 80 mg, cupric oxide 2 mg, β-carotene 15 mg, vitamin C 500 mg, and vitamin E 400 IU taken in divided doses bid reduces risk of progression (eg, *Ocuvite PreserVision*).

Diabetic Retinopathy: Glycemic control (see p 54)

Glaucoma: Treat when pressures are > 25 mm Hg or with optic nerve damage or visual field loss (see **Table 76**). Instill drops, close eye for 3–5 min to reduce systemic absorption.

Table 76. Agents for Treating Glaucoma			
Drug	**Strength**	**Dosage**	**Comments (Metabolism)**
Adrenergic Agonists (bottles with purple caps)			
Apraclonidine (*Iopidine*)	0.5%, 1%	1–2 drops tid	Low BP, fatigue, drowsiness, dry mouth, dry nose (unknown)
Brimonidine (*Alphagan*)	0.2%	1 drop tid	Low BP, fatigue, drowsiness, dry mouth, dry nose (L)
(*Alphagan P*)	0.15%	1 drop tid	Benzalkonium-chloride free
Dipivefrin (*AKPro, Propine*)	0.1%	1 drop bid	HTN, headache, tachycardia, arrhythmia (eye, L)
Epinephrine (*Epifrin, Glaucon*)	0.1%–2%	1 drop qd–bid	HTN, headache, tachycardia, arrhythmia (L)
Epinephrine borate (*Epinal*)	0.25%–0.5%	1 drop bid	HTN, headache, tachycardia, arrhythmia (L)
β-Blockers (bottles with blue or yellow caps)			Class side effects: hypotension, bradycardia, CHF, bronchospasm, anxiety, confusion, hallucination, diarrhea, nausea, cramps, lethargy, weakness, masking of hypoglycemia, impotence (L)
Betaxolol (*Betoptic, Betoptic-S*)	0.25%, 0.5%	1–2 drops bid	
Carteolol (*Ocupress*)	1%	1 drop bid	
Levobunolol (*AKBeta, Betagan*)	0.25%, 0.5%	1 drop bid	
Metipranolol (*OptiPranolol*)	0.3%	1 drop bid	
Timolol drops (*Betimol, Timoptic*)	0.25%, 0.5%	1 drop bid	
Timolol gel (*Timoptic–XE*)	0.25%, 0.5%	1 drop qd (in AM)	
Miotics, Direct-Acting (bottles with green caps)			
Pilocarpine gel (*Pilopine HS*)	4%	1/2" qhs	Systemic cholinergic effects (tissues, K)
(*Ocusert*)	20, 40 μg/h	Weekly	

Table 76. Agents for Treating Glaucoma (cont.)

Drug	Strength	Dosage	Comments (Metabolism)
Pilocarpine (*Adsorbocarpine, Akarpine, Isopto Carpine, Pilagan, Pilocar, Piloptic, Pilostat*)	0.25%–10%	1 drop qid	Systemic cholinergic effects are rare (K)
Miotics, Cholinesterase Inhibitors (bottles with green caps)			Class side effects: cholinomimetic effects (sweating, tremor, headache, salivation), confusion, high or low BP, bradycardia, bronchoconstriction, urinary frequency, cramps, diarrhea, nausea, deterioration of mental status in persons with AD
Demecarium (*Humorsol*)	0.125%, 0.25%	1–2 drops bid	
Echothiophate (*Phospholine*)	0.03%–0.25%	1 drop bid	
Isoflurophate (*Floropryl*)	0.025%	0.25"/8–72 h	
Physostigmine (*Eserine, Fisostin, Isopto Eserine*)	0.25% ointment	1" tid	(L)
Carbonic Anhydrase Inhibitors (bottles with orange caps)			
Topical			Caution in renal failure (K)
√ Brinzolamide (*Azopt*)	1%	1 drop tid	
√ Dorzolamide (*Trusopt*)	2%	1 drop tid	
Oral			Class side effects: fatigue, weight loss, paresthesias, depression, COPD exacerbation, cramps, diarrhea, renal failure, blood dyscrasias, hypokalemia, acidosis; not recommended in renal failure (K)
Acetazolamide (eg, *Diamox*)	125–500 mg, 500 mg SR	250–500 mg bid–qid, 500 SR bid	
Dichlorphenamide (*Daranide*)	50 mg	25–50 mg qd–tid	
Methazolamide (eg, *Neptazane*)	25–50 mg	50–100 mg bid–tid	(L,K)
Prostaglandin Analogues			Class side effects: change in eye color and periorbital tissues, hyperemia, itching; expensive (K, L)
Bimatoprost (*Lumigan*)	0.03%	1 drop hs	(L,K,F)
Latanoprost (*Xalatan*)	0.005%	1 drop hs	(L)
Travoprost (*Travatan*)	0.004%	1 drop hs	(L)
Unoprostone (*Rescula*)	0.15%	1 drop hs	(L)
Other topical			
Dorzolamide/timolol (*Cosopt*)	0.2%, 0.05%	1 drop bid	Unusual taste, ocular itching, burning (K, L)

Note: Patients may not know names of drugs but instead refer to them by the color of the bottle cap. The usual color scheme is referenced above. √ = preferred for treating older persons.

Low-Vision Rehabilitation and Aids

Refer patients with uncompensated visual loss causing functional deficits. Aids include optical, nonoptical, low- and high-technology devices. Strategies include improved illumination, increased contrast, magnification, and auditory and tactile feedback. Environmental modifications include using color contrast, floor lamps to reduce glare, motion sensors to turn on lights, high-technology options including video magnification with closed-circuit television and word processing programs to enlarge text.

Acute Conjunctivitis

Symptoms: Red eye, foreign body sensation, discharge, photophobia

Signs: Conjunctival hyperemia and discharge. Visual acuity, pupillary light reflexes, and visual fields are normal. If eye functions are abnormal, refer to ophthalmology for urgent diagnosis.

Differential diagnosis: Acute iritis, acute glaucoma, episcleritis, or scleritis.

Etiology: Viral, bacterial, chlamydial, chemical, foreign body

Viral versus bacterial: **Viral**—profuse tearing, minimal exudation, preauricular adenopathy common, monocytes in stained scrapings and exudates; **bacterial**—moderate tearing, profuse exudation, preauricular adenopathy uncommon, bacteria and polymorphonuclear cells in stained scrapings and exudates; **both**—minimal itching, generalized hyperemia, occasional sore throat and fever.

Treatment: Majority are viral; treat symptoms with artificial tears and cool compresses. If purulent discharge, suspect bacterial; start broad-spectrum topical antibiotics (see **Table 77**). If severe, obtain culture and Gram's stain, then start treatment. If signs and symptoms fail to improve in 24–48 h, refer to ophthalmologist. If vision decreased or severe pain, refer to ophthalmologist immediately.

Other: Frequent hand washing and use of separate towels to avoid spread

Table 77. Treatment for Acute Bacterial Conjunctivitis*		
Agent	**Formulations****	**Comment**
Ciprofloxacin (*Ciloxan Ophthalmic*)	0.3% sol, 0.3% oint	Very broad spectrum, well tolerated, a 1st choice in severe cases, expensive
Erythromycin ophthalmic (*AK-Mycin, Ilotycin*)	5 mg/gm oint	Good if staphylococcal blepharitis is present
Norfloxacin (*Chibroxin*)	0.3% sol	Very broad spectrum, well tolerated, a 1st choice in severe cases, expensive
Ofloxacin (*Floxin, Ocuflox Ophthalmic*)	0.3% sol, 0.3% oint	Very broad spectrum, well tolerated, a 1st choice in severe cases, expensive
Sulfacetamide sodium (*Sodium Sulamyd*)	10%, 30% drops, 10% oint	Same coverage as trimethoprim and polymyxin
Tobramycin (*AKTob, Tobrex*)	3 mg/gm oint, 3 mg/mL sol	Well tolerated, but more corneal toxic
Trimethoprim and polymyxin (*Polytrim*)	1 mg/mL, 10,000 IU/mL sol	Well tolerated but some gaps in coverage

* Do not use steroid or steroid-antibiotic preparations in initial treatment.

** In mild cases solution is applied qid and gel or ointments bid for 5–7 d. In more severe cases solution is applied q 2–3 h, ointment qid; as the eye improves, solution is applied qid and ointment, bid.

PREVENTION (See also p 132)
- Annual breast and pelvic and perineal examination
- Annual mammography as appropriate
- Discuss HRT risks/benefits with patients on treatment
- One negative Pap smear after 65 yr if low risk (ie, single established sexual partner, good prior screening, no hx of abnormal Pap smear)
- Osteoporosis evaluation (see p 112)

COMMON DISORDERS
Vulvar Diseases
Non-neoplastic:
- Lichen sclerosus—Occurs commonly on vulva of middle-aged and older women; causes 1/3 of benign vulvar lesions, extends to perirectal areas (classic hourglass appearance); lesions are white to pink macules or papules, may coalesce; symptoms are none or itching, soreness, or dyspareunia. Must biopsy for diagnosis: Associated with squamous cell cancer in 4% to 5%. R_x: Clobetasol propionate 0.05% qd–bid for 8–12 wk; then taper gradually to zero. Long-term follow-up advised.
- Squamous hyperplasia—Raised white keratinized lesions difficult to distinguish from vulvar intraepithelial neoplasia (VIN); must biopsy to exclude malignancy. R_x: Betamethasone dipropionate 0.05% for 6–8 wk, then 1% hydrocortisone if symptoms persist; long term follow-up advised.

Neoplastic:
- VIN—Most often seen in postmenopausal women; asymptomatic or may cause pruritus; appear as hypo- or hyperpigmented keratinized lesions; often multifocal; inspection ± colposcopy of the entire vulva with biopsy of most worrisome lesions; lesions graded on degree of atypia. R_x: surgical or other ablative therapy.
- Vulvar malignancy—Half of cases occur in women aged > 70 yr; 80% are squamous cell, with melanoma, sarcoma, basal cell, and adenocarcinoma < 20%; biopsy any suspicious lesion. R_x: radical surgery is preferred treatment.

Postmenopausal Bleeding
Bleeding after 1 yr of amenorrhea:
- Exclude malignancy, identify source, treat symptoms.
- Examine genitalia, perineum, rectum.
- If endometrial source, use endometrial biopsy or vaginal probe ultrasound to assess endometrial thickness (< 5 mm virtually excludes malignancy).
- D&C when endometrium not otherwise adequately assessed.
- Women on combination continuous estrogen and progesterone who bleed after 12 mo need evaluation.
- Those on cyclic replacement with bleeding at unexpected times (ie, bleeding other than during the second week of progesterone therapy) need evaluation.
- Women on unopposed estrogen who bleed at any time need evaluation.

Hot Flushes
- Vasomotor symptoms respond to estrogen (see **Table 78**) in dose-response fashion; start low dose, titrate to effect.

- If estrogen cannot be taken, try one of the less effective alternatives:
  - megestrol (*Megace*): [T: 20, 40] 20 mg qd-bid
  - venlafaxine 75 mg/d; paroxetine 20 mg/d
  - clonidine (*Catapres, Duraclon*): [T: 0.1, 0.2, 0.3] 0.1–0.3 mg/d; use lowest effective dose, watch for orthostatic ↓ BP and rebound ↑ BP if used intermittently

Vaginal Prolapse

- Child-bearing and other causes of increased intra-abdominal pressure weaken connective tissue and muscles supporting the genital organs, leading to prolapse.
- Symptoms include: Pelvic pressure, back pain, fecal or urinary incontinence, difficulty evacuating the rectum. Symptoms may be present even with mild prolapse.
- The degree of prolapse and organs involved dictate therapy; no therapy if asymptomatic.
- Estrogen and Kegel's exercises may help in mild cases.
- Pessary or surgery indicated with greater symptoms. Surgery needed for 4th-degree symptomatic prolapse.
- Precise anatomic defect(s) dictates the surgical approach.
- A common (ACOG) classification for degrees of prolapse:
  - First degree—extension to mid-vagina
  - Second degree—approaching hymenal ring
  - Third degree—at hymenal ring
  - Fourth degree—beyond hymenal ring

Atrophic Vaginitis (See p 154)

HORMONE REPLACEMENT THERAPY
Estrogen Replacement

Combined hormone (estrogen and progesterone) therapy is associated with increased risk of MI, PE, stroke, and breast cancer. Combined therapy is associated with reduced risk of hip fracture and colorectal cancer. The effects of unopposed estrogen on these outcomes are uncertain, but unopposed estrogen is associated with increased risk of endometrial cancer. Other risks of estrogen therapy include gallbladder disease and possibly ovarian cancer. Positive effects on urogenital health include reduced vaginal dryness, reduced dyspareunia, reduction in recurrent urinary tract infections, and possibly maintenance of continence.

- When the patient has a uterus, estrogen should be combined with progesterone to reduce endometrial cancer risk.
- Some women prefer unopposed estrogen and annual endometrial biopsy.
- Common regimens are given in **Table 78**.
- Older women can get hot flushes as a result of sudden discontinuation of estrogen. A tapering regimen (eg, qod for 1–2 months and then q3d for a few months) may be beneficial.

Contraindications:
- Undiagnosed vaginal bleeding
- Thromboembolic disease
- Breast cancer
- Endometrial cancer greater than stage 1
- Possibly gallbladder disease
- Menstrual migraine

Table 78. Common Regimens for Hormone Replacement Therapy				
Preparation	Starting Dosage (mg/d)	Cyclic Dosing	Continuous Dosing	Formulations
Conjugated equine estrogen (*Premarin*)*	0.3–0.625	—	Daily	[T: 0.3, 0.625, 0.9, 1.25, 2.5]
Conjugated synthetic estrogen (*Cenestin*)	0.625	—	Daily	[T: 0.625, 0.9, 1.25]
Esterified estrogen (eg, *Estratab, Menest*)*	0.3–0.625	—	Daily	[T: 0.3, 0.625, 1.25, 2.5]
Estropipate (*Ogen, Ortho-Est*)*	0.625	—	Daily	[T: 0.625, 1.25, 2.5]
Micronized 17-β estradiol (*Estrace*)*	0.5–1.0	—	Daily	[T: 0.5, 1, 2]
Transdermal estrogen				
(*Alora*)	0.05–0.75	—	Biweekly	[0.05 0.075, 0.1]
(*Estraderm*)*	0.05–0.75		Biweekly	[0.05, 0.1]
(*Vivelle*)*	0.0375–0.05		Biweekly	[0.025, 0.0375, 0.05, 0.075, 0.1]
(*Climara*)*	0.025–0.05	—	Weekly	[0.025, 0.05, 0.075, 0.1]
(*FemPatch*)	0.025–0.05		Weekly	[0.025]
Estradiol *and* norethindrone (*CombiPatch*)	0.05/0.14	Biweekly for 3 wk, 1wk off	—	[0.05/0.14, 0.05/0.25]
Medroxyprogesterone (*Cycrin, Provera*)	2.5–10.0	5–10 mg, days 1–14	2.5–5 mg daily	[T: 2.5, 5, 10]
Combinations				
Conjugated estrogen *and* medroxyprogesterone (*Prempro*)	0.625 2.5, 5.0	—	Daily	[Fixed dose 0.625/2.5 or 0.625/5.0]
Conjugated estrogen *and* medroxyprogesterone (*Premphase*)	0.625 5.0	Days 1–28 Days 15–28	—	[Fixed dose 0.625 days 1–14, 0.625/5.0 days 15–28]
Estradiol *and* norethindrone (*FEMHRT 1/5*)	1.0 5.0	—	Daily	[Fixed dose 1.0/5.0]

* FDA approved for long-term use to prevent osteoporosis.

ASSESSMENT INSTRUMENTS

MINI-COG ASSESSMENT INSTRUMENT FOR DEMENTIA

The Mini-Cog assessment instrument combines an uncued 3-item recall test with a clock-drawing test (CDT). The Mini-Cog can be administered in about 3 minutes, requires no special equipment, and is relatively uninfluenced by level of education or language variations.

Administration

The test is administered as follows:

1. Instruct the patient to listen carefully to and remember 3 unrelated words and then to repeat the words.
2. Instruct the patient to draw the face of a clock, either on a blank sheet of paper, or on a sheet with the clock circle already drawn on the page. After the patient puts the numbers on the clock face, ask him or her to draw the hands of the clock to read a specific time, such as 11:20. These instructions can be repeated, but no additional instructions should be given. Give the patient as much time as needed to complete the task. The CDT serves as the recall distractor.
3. Ask the patient to repeat the 3 previously presented words.

Scoring

Give 1 point for each recalled word after the CDT distractor. Score 1–3.
   - A score of 0 indicates positive screen for dementia.
   - A score of 1 or 2 with an abnormal CDT indicates positive screen for dementia.
   - A score of 1 or 2 with a normal CDT indicates negative screen for dementia.
   - A score of 3 indicates negative screen for dementia.
The CDT is considered normal if all numbers are present in the correct sequence and position, and the hands readably display the requested time.

Source: Borson S, Scanlan J, Brush M, Vitaliano P, Dokmak A. The mini-cog: a cognitive "vital signs" measure for dementia screening in multi-lingual elderly. *Int J Geriatr Psychiatry* 2000; 15(11): 1021–1027.

PHYSICAL SELF-MAINTENANCE SCALE (ACTIVITIES OF DAILY LIVING, OR ADLs

In each category, circle the item that most closely describes the person's highest level of functioning and record the score assigned to that level (either 1 or 0) in the blank at the beginning of the category.

A. Toilet _____
1. Care for self at toilet completely; no incontinence 1
2. Needs to be reminded, or needs help in cleaning self, or has rare
   (weekly at most) accidents 0
3. Soiling or wetting while asleep more than once a week 0
4. Soiling or wetting while awake more than once a week 0
5. No control of bowels or bladder 0

B. Feeding
1. Eats without assistance 1
2. Eats with minor assistance at meal times and/or with special
   preparation of food, or help in cleaning up after meals 0
3. Feeds self with moderate assistance and is untidy 0
4. Requires extensive assistance for all meals 0
5. Does not feed self at all and resists efforts of others to feed him or her 0

C. Dressing
1. Dresses, undresses, and selects clothes from own wardrobe 1
2. Dresses and undresses self, with minor assistance 0
3. Needs moderate assistance in dressing and selection of clothes. 0
4. Needs major assistance in dressing, but cooperates with efforts of
   others to help 0
5. Completely unable to dress self and resists efforts of others to help 0

D. Grooming (neatness, hair, nails, hands, face, clothing)
1. Always neatly dressed, well-groomed, without assistance 1
2. Grooms self adequately with occasional minor assistance, eg, with shaving 0
3. Needs moderate and regular assistance or supervision with grooming 0
4. Needs total grooming care, but can remain well-groomed after help from others 0
5. Actively negates all efforts of others to maintain grooming 0

E. Physical Ambulation
1. Goes about grounds or city 1
2. Ambulates within residence on or about one block distant 0
3. Ambulates with assistance of (check one)
   a ( ) another person, b ( ) railing, c ( ) cane, d ( ) walker, e ( ) wheelchair 0
   1.___Gets in and out without help. 2.___Needs help getting in and out
4. Sits unsupported in chair or wheelchair, but cannot propel self without help 0
5. Bedridden more than half the time 0

F. Bathing
1. Bathes self (tub, shower, sponge bath) without help. 1
2. Bathes self with help getting in and out of tub. 0
3. Washes face and hands only, but cannot bathe rest of body 0
4. Does not wash self, but is cooperative with those who bathe him or her. 0
5. Does not try to wash self and resists efforts to keep him or her clean. 0

For scoring interpretation and source, see note following the next instrument.

INSTRUMENTAL ACTIVITIES OF DAILY LIVING SCALE (IADLs)

In each category, circle the item that most closely describes the person's highest level
of functioning and record the score assigned to that level (either 1 or 0) in the blank at
the beginning of the category.

A. Ability to Use Telephone
1. Operates telephone on own initiative; looks up and dials numbers. 1
2. Dials a few well-known numbers. 1
3. Answers telephone, but does not dial. 1
4. Does not use telephone at all. 0

B. Shopping
1. Takes care of all shopping needs independently. 1
2. Shops independently for small purchases. 0
3. Needs to be accompanied on any shopping trip. 0
4. Completely unable to shop. 0

C. **Food Preparation** _____

  1. Plans, prepares, and serves adequate meals independently. 1

  2. Prepares adequate meals if supplied with ingredients. 0

  3. Heats and serves prepared meals or prepares meals, but does not
     maintain adequate diet. 0

  4. Needs to have meals prepared and served. 0

D. **Housekeeping** _____

  1. Maintains house alone or with occasional assistance (eg, heavy-
     work domestic help). 1

  2. Performs light daily tasks such as dishwashing, bedmaking. 1

  3. Performs light daily tasks, but cannot maintain acceptable level of
     cleanliness. 1

  4. Needs help with all home maintenance tasks. 1

  5. Does not participate in any housekeeping tasks. 0

E. **Laundry** _____

  1. Does personal laundry completely. 1

  2. Launders small items; rinses socks, stockings, etc. 1

  3. All laundry must be done by others. 0

F. **Mode of Transportation** _____

  1. Travels independently on public transportation or drives own car. 1

  2. Arranges own travel via taxi, but does not otherwise use public
     transportation. 1

  3. Travels on public transportation when assisted or accompanied
     by another. 1

  4. Travel limited to taxi or automobile with assistance of another. 0

  5. Does not travel at all. 0

G. **Responsibility for Own Medications** _____

  1. Is responsible for taking medication in correct dosages at correct time. 1

  2. Takes responsibility if medication is prepared in advance in separate
     dosages. 0

  3. Is not capable of dispensing own medication. 0

H. **Ability to Handle Finances** _____

  1. Manages financial matters independently (budgets, writes checks,
     pays rent and bills, goes to bank); collects and keeps track of income. 1

  2. Manages day-to-day purchases, but needs help with banking,
     major purchases, etc. 1

  3. Incapable of handling money. 0

Scoring Interpretation: For ADLs, the total score ranges from 0 to 6, and for IADLs, from 0 to 8. In some categories, only the highest level of function receives a 1; in others, two or more levels have scores of 1 because each describes competence that represents some minimal level of function. These screens are useful for indicating specifically how a person is performing at the present time. When they are also used over time, they serve as documentation of a person's functional improvement or deterioration.

Source: Republished with permission from Lawton MP, Brody EM. Assessment of older people: self-maintaining and instrumental activities of daily living. _Gerontologist_ 1969, 9:179–186. Permission conveyed through Copyright Clearance Center, Inc.

GERIATRIC DEPRESSION SCALE (GDS, SHORT FORM)

Choose the best answer for how you felt over the past week.

1. Are you basically satisfied with your life?	yes/**no**
2. Have you dropped many of your activities and interests?	**yes**/no
3. Do you feel that your life is empty?	**yes**/no
4. Do you often get bored?	**yes**/no

5. Are you in good spirits most of the time? yes/**no**
6. Are you afraid that something bad is going to happen to you? **yes**/no
7. Do you feel happy most of the time? yes/**no**
8. Do you often feel helpless? **yes**/no
9. Do you prefer to stay at home, rather than going out and doing new things? **yes**/no
10. Do you feel you have more problems with memory than most? **yes**/no
11. Do you think it is wonderful to be alive now? yes/**no**
12. Do you feel pretty worthless the way you are now? **yes**/no
13. Do you feel full of energy? yes/**no**
14. Do you feel that your situation is hopeless? **yes**/no
15. Do you think that most people are better off than you are? **yes**/no

Score 1 point for each bolded answer. Cut-off: normal (0–5), above 5 suggests depression.

Source: Courtesy of Jerome A. Yesavage, MD. For 30 translations of the GDS, see
http://www.stanford.edu/~yesavage/GDS.html
For additional information on administration and scoring refer to the following references:
1. Sheikh JI, Yesavage JA. Geriatric Depression Scale: recent evidence and development of a shorter version. *Clin Gerontol.* 1986;5:165–172.
2. Feher EP, Larrabee GJ, Crook TH 3rd. Factors attenuating the validity of the Geriatric Depression Scale in a dementia population. *J Am Geriatr Soc.* 1992;40:906–909.
3. Yesavage JA, Brink TL, Rose TL, et al. Development and validation of a geriatric depression rating scale: a preliminary report. *J Psychiatr Res.* 1983;17:27.

BRIEF HEARING LOSS SCREENER

Points

1. Age:_____ _____
 If age > 70 years = 1 point
2. Sex: Male_____ Female_____ _____
 If male = 1 point
3. Highest grade attended: _____
 12th grade or less _____
 higher than 12th grade_____
 If ≤ 12th grade = 1 point
4. Have you ever had deafness or trouble hearing with one or both ears? ____0____
 Yes_____, continue to Question #5.
 No_____, go to Question #6.
 No points assigned to this question.
5. Did you ever see a doctor about it? _____
 Yes_____No_____
 If "Yes" = 2 points
6. Without a hearing aid, can you usually hear and understand what a person _____
 says without seeing his/her face if that person whispers to you
 from across the room?
 Yes_____No_____
 If "No" = 1 point
7. Without a hearing aid, can you usually hear and understand what a person _____
 says without seeing his/her face if that person talks to you in a normal voice
 from across the room?
 Yes_____No_____
 If "No" = 2 points

TOTAL _____

3 or more points is a positive score indicating the need for further evaluation.

Test Characteristics of This Screener With Established Hearing Loss Criteria

	Sensitivity	Specificity	Pos Predictive Value	Neg Predictive Value
Ventry-Weinstein criteria	80%	80%	45%	95%
High-frequency pure-tone average	59%	88%	76%	77%

Source: Reuben DB, Walsh K, Moore AA, et al. Hearing loss in community-dwelling older persons: national prevalence data and identification using simple questions. *J Am Geriatr Soc.* 1998;46:1011. Reprinted with permission.

PERFORMANCE-ORIENTED MOBILITY ASSESSMENT (POMA)

Balance

Chair: Instructions: Place a hard armless chair against a wall. The following maneuvers are tested.

1. Sitting down
   0 = unable without help or collapses (plops) into chair *or* lands off center of chair
   1 = able and does not meet criteria for 0 or 2
   2 = sits in a smooth, safe motion *and* ends with buttocks against back of chair and thighs centered on chair
2. Sitting balance
   0 = unable to maintain position (marked slide forward or leans forward or to side)
   1 = eans in chair slightly or slight increased distance from buttocks to back of chair
   2 = steady, safe, upright
3. Arising
   0 = unable without help or loses balance or requires > three attempts
   1 = able but requires three attempts
   2 = able in ≤ two attempts
4. Immediate standing balance (first 5 seconds)
   0 = unsteady, marked staggering, moves feet, marked trunk sway or grabs object for support
   1 = steady but uses walker or cane or mild staggering but catches self without grabbing object
   2 = steady without walker or cane or other support

Stand

5a. Side-by-side standing balance
   0 = unable *or* unsteady *or* holds ≤ 3 seconds
   1 = able *but* uses cane, walker, or other support *or* holds for 4–9 seconds
   2 = narrow stance without support for 10 seconds
5b. Timing ___ . ___ seconds
6. Pull test (person at maximum position attained in #5, examiner stands behind and exerts mild pull back at waist)
   0 = begins to fall
   1 = takes more than two steps back
   2 = fewer than two steps backward and steady
7a. Able to stand on right leg unsupported
   0 = unable *or* holds onto any objects *or* able for < 3 seconds
   1 = able for 3 or 4 seconds
   2 = able for 5 seconds
7b. Timing ___ . ___ seconds

8a. Able to stand on left leg unsupported
    0 = unable *or* holds onto any object *or* able for < 3 seconds
    1 = able for 3 or 4 seconds
    2 = able for 5 seconds
8b. Timing __ __ . __ seconds
9a. Semitandem stand
    0 = unable to stand with one foot half in front of other with feet touching *or*
        begins to fall *or* holds for ≤ 3 seconds
    1 = able for 4 to 9 seconds
    2 = able to semitandem stand for 10 seconds
9b. Timing __ __ . __ seconds
10a. Tandem stand
    0 = unable to stand with one foot in front of other *or* begins to fall *or* holds for
        ≤ 3 seconds
    1 = able for 4 to 9 seconds
    2 = able to tandem stand for 10 seconds
10b. Timing __ __ . __ seconds
11. Bending over (to pick up a pen off floor)
    0 = unable *or* is unsteady
    1 = able, but requires more than one attempt to get up
    2 = able and is steady
12. Toe stand
    0 = unable
    1 = able but < 3 seconds
    2 = able for 3 seconds
13. Heel stand
    0 = unable
    1 = able but < 3 seconds
    2 = able for 3 seconds

Gait: Instructions: Person stands with examiner, walks down 10-ft walkway (measured). Ask the person to walk down walkway, turn, and walk back. The person should use customary walking aid.

Bare Floor (flat, even surface)
1. Type of surface: 1 = linoleum or tile; 2 = wood; 3 = cement or concrete; 4 = other
    _____ [not included in scoring]
2. Initiation of gait (immediately after told to "go")
    0 = any hesitancy or multiple attempts to start
    1 = no hesitancy
3. Path (estimated in relation to tape measure). Observe excursion of foot closest to tape
    measure over middle 8 feet of course.
    0 = marked deviation
    1 = mild or moderate deviation *or* uses walking aid
    2 = straight without walking aid
4. Missed step (trip or loss of balance)
    0 = yes, and would have fallen *or* more than two missed steps
    1 = yes, but appropriate attempt to recover *and* no more than two missed steps
    2 = none
5. Turning (while walking)
    0 = almost falls
    1 = mild staggering, but catches self, uses walker or cane
    2 = steady, without walking aid
6. Step over obstacles (to be assessed in a separate walk with two shoes placed on course
    4 feet apart)
    0 = begins to fall at any obstacle *or* unable *or* walks around any obstacle *or* > two
        missed steps

1 = able to step over all obstacles, but some staggering and catches self *or* one
to two missed steps

2 = able and steady at stepping over all four obstacles with no missed steps

Source: Courtesy of Mary E. Tinetti, MD. Adapted with permission.

ABNORMAL INVOLUNTARY MOVEMENT SCALE (AIMS)

Examination Procedure

Either before or after completing the examination procedure, observe the patient
unobtrusively, at rest (eg, in waiting room). The chair to be used in this examination
should be a hard, firm one without arms.

1. Ask patient to remove shoes and socks.
2. Ask patient whether there is anything in his/her mouth (ie, gum, candy, etc) and if
   there is, to remove it.
3. Ask patient about the **current** condition of his/her teeth. Ask patient if he/she wears
   dentures. Do teeth or dentures bother patient **now**?
4. Ask patient whether he/she notices any movements in mouth, face, hands, or feet. If
   yes, ask to describe and to what extent they **currently** bother patient or interfere
   with his/her activities.
5. Have patient sit in chair with hands on knees, legs slightly apart, and feet flat on
   floor. (Look at entire body for movements while in this position.)
6. Ask patient to sit with hands hanging unsupported. If male, between legs, if female
   and wearing a dress, hanging over knees. (Observe hands and other body areas.)
7. Ask patient to open mouth. (Observe tongue at rest within mouth.) Do this twice.
8. Ask patient to protrude tongue. (Observe abnormalities of tongue movement.) Do this
   twice.
9. Ask patient to tap thumb with each finger as rapidly as possible for 10–15 seconds;
   separately with right hand, then with left hand. (Observe facial and leg movements.)
10. Flex and extend patient's left and right arms (one at a time). (Note any rigidity.)
11. Ask patient to stand up. (Observe in profile. Observe all body areas again, hips
    included.)
12. Ask patient to extend both arms outstretched in front with palms down. (Observe
    trunk, legs, and mouth.)
13. Have patient walk a few paces, turn, and walk back to chair. (Observe hands and
    gait.) Do this twice.

Instructions: Complete examination procedure before making ratings. Rate highest
severity observed.
Code:
   1 None
   2 Minimal, may be extreme normal
   3 Mild
   4 Moderate
   5 Severe

AIMS

Facial and Oral Movements

1. Muscles of facial expression (eg, movements of forehead, eyebrows, periorbital area, cheeks; including frowning, blinking, smiling, grimacing)

    1   2   3   4   5

2. Lips and perioral area (eg, puckering, pouting, smacking)

    1   2   3   4   5

3. Jaw (eg, biting, clenching, chewing, mouth opening, lateral movement)

    1   2   3   4   5

4. Tongue (rate only increase in movement both in and out of mouth, NOT inability to sustain movement)

    1   2   3   4   5

Extremity Movements

5. Upper (arms, wrists, hands, fingers). Include choreic movements (ie, rapid, objectively purposeless, irregular, spontaneous), athetoid movements (ie, slow, irregular, complex, serpentine). Do NOT include tremor (ie, repetitive, regular, rhythmic).

    1   2   3   4   5

6. Lower (legs, knees, ankles, toes). (Eg, lateral knee movement, foot tapping, heel dropping, foot squirming, inversion and eversion of foot)

    1   2   3   4   5

Trunk Movements

7. Neck, shoulders, hips (eg, rocking, twisting, squirming, pelvic gyrations)

    1   2   3   4   5

Global Judgments

8. Severity of abnormal movements
   1 None, normal
   2 Minimal
   3 Mild
   4 Moderate
   5 Severe

9. Incapacitation due to abnormal movements
   1 None, normal
   2 Minimal
   3 Mild
   4 Moderate
   5 Severe

10. Patient's awareness of abnormal movements (rate only patient's report)
   1 No awareness
   2 Aware, no distress
   3 Aware, mild distress
   4 Aware, moderate distress
   5 Aware, severe distress

Dental Status

11. Current problems with teeth and/or dentures
    1 No
    2 Yes
12. Does patient usually wear dentures?
    1 No
    2 Yes

Source: Adapted from Department of Health and Human Services, Public Health Service, Alcohol, Drug Abuse and Mental Health Administration, National Institute of Mental Health. *Treatment Strategies in Schizophrenia Study*. ADM-117. Revised 1985.

PAIN SCALES FOR ASSESSING PAIN INTENSITY

Use copies of pain scales that are large enough for older patients to see comfortably (14-point font or larger).

Faces Pain Scale

Place an X under the face that best represents the severity or intensity of your pain right now.

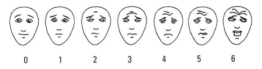

Source: Reprinted from *Pain*, 41(2), Bien D, Reeve R, Champion G, et al. The Faces Pain Scale for the self-assessment of the severity of pain experienced by children: development and initial validation, and preliminary investigation for ratio scale properties. 139–150, Copyright 1990, with permission from Elsevier Science.

0–10 Numeric Rating Scales

Verbal: On a scale of 0–10, with 0 being no pain and 10 being the most intense pain imaginable, what would you rate the severity or intensity of your pain right now? _____

Source: Keela Herr, 1999.

Visual: Circle the number that best represents the severity or intensity of your pain right now.

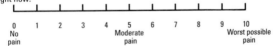

Source: Carr DB, Jacox AK, Chapman CR, et al. *Acute Pain Management: Operative Medical Procedures and Trauma*. Clinical Practice Guideline No. 1. Rockville, MD: AHCPR, Public Health Service, US Dept of Health and Human Services; February 1992. AHCPR Publication No. 92-0032.

Verbal Descriptor Scale

Place an X beside the words that best describe the severity or intensity of your pain right now. Mark one set of words.

——The Most Intense Pain Imaginable
——Very Severe Pain
——Severe Pain
——Moderate Pain
——Mild Pain
——Slight Pain
——No Pain

Source: Keela Herr, 1999.

References

AGS Panel on Persistent Pain in Older Persons. The management of persistent pain in older persons. *J Am Geriatr Soc.* 2002; 50(6, Suppl): S205–S224.

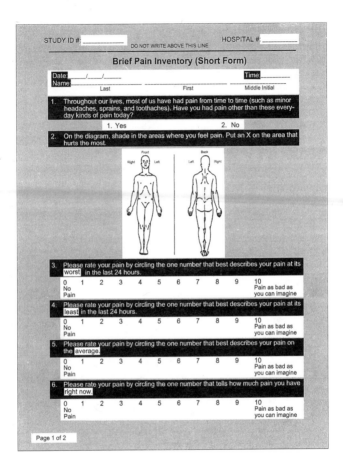

STUDY ID #: _____ HOSPITAL #: _____

DO NOT WRITE ABOVE THIS LINE

Brief Pain Inventory (Short Form)

Date: ___/___/___ Time: _____

Name: _____

Last   First   Middle Initial

1. Throughout our lives, most of us have had pain from time to time (such as minor headaches, sprains, and toothaches). Have you had pain other than these every-day kinds of pain today?

      1. Yes   2. No

2. On the diagram, shade in the areas where you feel pain. Put an X on the area that hurts the most.

3. Please rate your pain by circling the one number that best describes your pain at its **worst** in the last 24 hours.

0	1	2	3	4	5	6	7	8	9	10
No Pain										Pain as bad as you can imagine

4. Please rate your pain by circling the one number that best describes your pain at its **least** in the last 24 hours.

0	1	2	3	4	5	6	7	8	9	10
No Pain										Pain as bad as you can imagine

5. Please rate your pain by circling the one number that best describes your pain on the **average.**

0	1	2	3	4	5	6	7	8	9	10
No Pain										Pain as bad as you can imagine

6. Please rate your pain by circling the one number that tells how much pain you have **right now.**

0	1	2	3	4	5	6	7	8	9	10
No Pain										Pain as bad as you can imagine

Page 1 of 2

Date: ___/___/___

Time: _____

Name: _____

Last   First   Middle Initial

7. What treatments or medications are you receiving for your pain?

_____

_____

8. In the last 24 hours, how much relief have pain treatments or medications provided? Please circle the one percentage that most shows how much relief you have received.

0%	10%	20%	30%	40%	50%	60%	70%	80%	90%	100%
No Relief										Complete Relief

9. Circle the one number that describes how, during the past 24 hours, pain has interfered with your:

A. General Activity

0	1	2	3	4	5	6	7	8	9	10
Does not Interfere										Completely Interferes

B. Mood

0	1	2	3	4	5	6	7	8	9	10
Does not Interfere										Completely Interferes

C. Walking Ability

0	1	2	3	4	5	6	7	8	9	10
Does not Interfere										Completely Interferes

D. Normal Work (includes both work outside the home and housework)

0	1	2	3	4	5	6	7	8	9	10
Does not Interfere										Completely Interferes

E. Relations with other people

0	1	2	3	4	5	6	7	8	9	10
Does not Interfere										Completely Interferes

F. Sleep

0	1	2	3	4	5	6	7	8	9	10
Does not Interfere										Completely Interferes

G. Enjoyment of life

0	1	2	3	4	5	6	7	8	9	10
Does not Interfere										Completely Interferes

Page 2 of 2

Worst pain, or the arithmetic mean of the 4 severity items (items 3, 4, 5 & 6), can be used as measures of pain severity. The arithmetic mean of the 7 interference item (items 9A-G) can be used as a measure of pain interference. Scores on the BPI pain severity items are defined as mild (1–4), moderate (5–6), and severe (7–10). The tool can be used to follow the course of pain and response to interventions.

10-MINUTE SCREENER FOR GERIATRIC CONDITIONS

Problem	Screening Measure	Positive Screen
Vision	Two parts: Ask: "Do you have difficulty driving or watching television or reading or doing any of your daily activities because of your eyesight?" If yes, then: Test each eye with Snellen chart while patient wears corrective lenses (if applicable)	Yes to question and inability to read > 20/40 on Snellen chart
Hearing	Use audioscope set at 40 dB; test hearing using 1000 and 2000 Hz	Inability to hear 1000 or 2000 Hz in both ears, or inability to hear frequencies in either ear
Leg mobility	Time the patient after asking: "Rise from the chair. Walk 20 feet briskly, turn, walk back to the chair, and sit down."	Unable to complete task in 15 sec
Urinary incontinence	Two parts: Ask: "In the past year, have you ever lost your urine and gotten wet?" If yes, then ask: "Have you lost urine on at least 6 separate days?"	Yes to both questions
Nutrition, weight loss	Two parts Ask: "Have you lost 10 lb over the past 6 months without trying to do so?" Weigh the patient	Yes to the question or weight < 100 lb
Memory	Three-item recall	Unable to recall all items after 1 min
Depression	Ask: "Do you often feel sad or depressed?"	Yes to the question
Physical disability	Six questions: "Are you able to. . ." ". . .do strenuous activities like fast walking or bicycling?" ". . .do heavy work around the house, like washing windows, walls, or floors?" ". . .go shopping for groceries or clothes?" ". . .get to places out of walking distance?" ". . .bathe, either a sponge bath, tub bath, or shower?" ". . .dress, like putting on a shirt, buttoning and zipping, or putting on shoes?"	No to any of the questions

Source: Reprinted from *Am J Med*, 100, Moore AA, Siu AL, Screening for common problems in ambulatory elderly: clinical confirmation of a screen instrument, 440, Copyright 1998, with permission from Excerpta Medica, Inc.

AUA SYMPTOM INDEX FOR BPH

Questions to be answered (circle 1 number on each line)	Not at all	Less than 1 time in 5	Less than half the time	About half the time	More than half the time	Almost always
1. Over the past month or so, how often have you had a sensation of not emptying your bladder completely after you finished urinating?	0	1	2	3	4	5
2. Over the past month or so, how often have you had to urinate again less than two hours after you finished urinating?	0	1	2	3	4	5
3. Over the past month or so, how often have you found you stopped and started again several times when you urinated?	0	1	2	3	4	5
4. Over the past month or so, how often have you found it difficult to postpone urination?	0	1	2	3	4	5
5. Over the past month or so, how often have you had a weak urinary stream?	0	1	2	3	4	5
6. Over the past month or so, how often have you had to push or strain to begin urination?	0	1	2	3	4	5
7. Over the last month, how many times did you most typically get up to urinate from the time you went to bed at night until the time you got up in the morning?	(none) 0	(1 time) 1	(2 times) 2	(3 times) 3	(4 times) 4	(5 or more times) 5

AUA Symptom Score = sum of questions 1–7 = _____. For interpretation, see p 141.

Source: Barry MJ, Fowler FJ Jr, O'Leary MP et al. The American Urological Association symptom index for benign prostatic hyperplasia. *J Urol.* 1992;148(5):1549–1557. Reprinted with permission.

OBRA REGULATIONS

US Health Care Financing Administration (in 2001 renamed Centers for Medicare and Medicaid Services, or CMS) regulations regarding the use of certain medications in nursing homes are contained in the Omnibus Budget Reconciliation Act (OBRA) of 1987.

ANTIDEPRESSANT MEDICATIONS

Table 79. Recommended Maximum Doses of Antidepressants		
Drug	Usual Max Daily Dose (mg) for Age $\geq$ 65	Usual Max Daily Dose (mg)
Amitriptyline (*Elavil*)	150	300
Amoxapine (*Asendin*)	200	400
Desipramine (*Norpramin*)	150	300
Doxepin (*Adapin, Sinequan*)	150	300
Imipramine (*Tofranil*)	150	300
Maprotiline (*Ludiomil*)	150	300
Nortriptyline (*Aventyl, Pamelor*)	75	150
Protriptyline (*Vivactil*)	30	60
Trazodone (*Desyrel*)	300	600
Trimipramine (*Surmontil*)	150	300

ANTIPSYCHOTIC MEDICATIONS

Indications for appropriate use of antipsychotic medications are outlined in OBRA. In addition to psychotic disorders, these indications include specific nonpsychotic behavior associated with organic mental syndromes:

- Agitated psychotic symptoms (biting, kicking, scratching, assertive and belligerent behavior, sexual aggressiveness) that present a danger to themselves or others or interfere with family's and/or staff's ability to provide care (activities of daily living, or ADLs)
- Psychotic symptoms (hallucinations, delusions, paranoia)
- Continuous (24-h) crying out and screaming

Behavior less responsive to antipsychotic therapy includes:

- Repetitive, bothersome behavior (ie, pacing, wandering, repeated statements or words, calling out, fidgeting)
- Poor self-care
- Unsociability
- Indifference to surroundings
- Uncooperative behavior
- Restlessness
- Impaired memory
- Anxiety
- Depression
- Insomnia

If antipsychotic therapy is to be used for one or more of these symptoms only, then the use of antipsychotic agents is inappropriate. Because of their anticholinergic properties, antipsychotic agents may worsen these symptoms, especially symptoms of sedation and lethargy, as well as enhance "confusion."

Selection of an antipsychotic agent should be based on the side-effect profile since all antipsychotic agents are equally effective at equivalent doses. Coadministration of two or more antipsychotics does not have any pharmacologic basis or clinical advantage. Coadministration of two or more antipsychotic agents does not improve clinical response and increases the potential for side effects.

Once behavior control is obtained, assess patient to determine if precipitating event (stress from drugs, fluid or electrolyte changes, infection, changes in environment) has been resolved or patient has accommodated to the environment or situation. Determine whether the antipsychotic can be decreased in dose or tapered off completely by monitoring selected target symptoms for which the antipsychotic therapy was initiated. OBRA 1987 requires attempts at dose reduction within a 6-month period unless documented as to why this cannot be done. Identifying target symptoms is essential for adequate monitoring. Because of side effects, intermittent use (not prn) is preferable (ie, only when patient has behavior warranting use of these agents). For the recommended doses of antipsychotics, see **Table 80**.

Table 80. Recommended Maximum Doses of Antipsychotics			
Drug	Usual Max Daily Dose (mg) for Age ≥ 65	Usual Max Daily Dose (mg)	Daily Oral Dose (mg) for Residents with Organic Mental Syndromes
Acetophenazine (*Tindal*)	150	300	20
Chlorpromazine (*Thorazine*)	800	1600	75
Chlorprothixene (*Taractan*)	800	1600	75
Clozapine (*Clozaril*)	25	450	50
Fluphenazine (*Prolixin*)	20	40	4
Haloperidol (*Haldol*)	50	100	4
Loxapine (*Loxitane*)	125	250	10
Mesoridazine (*Serentil*)	250	500	25
Molindone (*Moban*)	112	225	10
Olanzapine (*Zyprexa*)	—	20	10
Quetiapine (*Seroquel*)	—	800	200
Perphenazine (*Trilafon*)	32	64	8
Promazine (*Sparine*)	50	500	150
Risperidone (*Risperdal*)	1	16	2
Thioridazine (*Mellaril*)	400	800	75
Thiothixene (*Navane*)	30	60	7
Trifluoperazine (*Stelazine*)	40	80	8
Triflupromazine (*Vesprin*)	100	20	—

ANXIOLYTIC MEDICATIONS

The use of anxiolytics is acceptable as long as other disease processes that could explain anxious behavior have been excluded. Daily use, at any dose, is for less than 4 continuous months, unless an attempt at dose reduction is unsuccessful. Proper indications include:
• Generalized anxiety disorder
• Organic mental syndrome (including dementia associated with agitation)
• Panic disorders
• Anxiety associated with other psychiatric disorder (eg, depression, adjustment disorder)

Table 81. Recommended Maximum Doses of Anxiolytics*		
Drug	Usual Daily Dose (mg) for Age ≥ 65	Usual Daily Dose (mg) for Age < 65
Alprazolam (*Xanax*)	2	4
Clorazepate (*Tranxene*)	30	60
Chlordiazepoxide (*Librium*)	40	100
Diazepam (*Valium*)	20	60
Halazepam (*Paxipam*)	80	160
Lorazepam (*Ativan*)	3	6
Meprobamate (*Miltown*)	600	1600
Oxazepam (*Serax*)	60	90
Prazepam (*Centrax*)	30	60

*CMS-OBRA guidelines strongly urge clinicians not to use barbiturates, glutethimide, and ethchlorvynol because of their side effects, pharmacokinetics, and addiction potential in the elderly person. Also, CMS discourages use of long-acting benzodiazepines in treating the elderly person.

HYPNOTIC MEDICATIONS

Hypnotics are allowed for 10 continuous days of use. If three unsuccessful attempts at dose reduction occur, then it is clinically contraindicated to reduce.

Table 82. Recommended Maximum Doses of Hypnotics*		
Drug	Usual Max Single Dose (mg) for Age ≥ 65	Usual Max Single Dose (mg)
Alprazolam (*Xanax*)	0.25	1.5
Amobarbital (*Amytal*)	150	300
Butabarbital (*Butisol*)	100	200
Chloral hydrate (*Noctec*)	750	1500
Chloral hydrate (*various*)	500	1000
Diphenhydramine (*Benadryl*)	25	50
Ethchlorvynol (*Placidyl*)	500	1000
Flurazepam (*Dalmane*)	15	30
Glutethimide (*Doriden*)	500	1000
Halazepam (*Paxipam*)	20	40
Hydroxyzine (*Atarax*)	50	100
Lorazepam (*Ativan*)	1	2
Methyprylon (*Noludar*)	200	400
Oxazepam (*Serax*)	15	30
Phenobarbital (*Nembutal*)	100	200
Secobarbital (*Seconal*)	100	200
Temazepam (*Restoril*)	15	30
Triazolam (*Halcion*)	0.125	0.5

*CMS-OBRA guidelines strongly urge clinicians not to use barbiturates, glutethimide, and ethchlorvynol because of their side effects, pharmacokinetics, and addiction potential in the elderly person. Also, CMS discourages use of long-acting benzodiazepines in treating the elderly person.

CMS CRITERIA: INAPPROPRIATE DRUG USE IN NURSING HOMES

On July 1, 1999, HCFA (the US Health Care Financing Administration, renamed in 2001 the Centers for Medicare and Medicaid Services, or CMS) modified its regulations regarding medication use by nursing home residents who are 65 years of age or older. As part of their review, surveyors will determine if the resident is taking any medications considered to have a high potential ("high severity") for severe adverse drug reactions (ADRs) or medications with a high potential for less severe ("low severity") ADRs. Residents receiving any medications will be monitored for ADRs. If an ADR is identified, the rationale for the medication use must be justified and considered appropriate. If it is not, a deficiency will be cited.

Persons wishing additional information are advised to contact the American Society of Consultant Pharmacists (see p 190 for telephone number, Web site).

The medications specified in **Table 83** are considered "high severity" by CMS and should be considered potentially inappropriate for use in treating elderly persons.

Table 83. Drugs Considered "High Severity" by CMS	
Class or Drug	**Comments**
Amitriptyline (*Elavil*)	May be used for neurogenic pain if an evaluation of risk vs. benefit of the drug is documented, including consideration of alternative therapies
Chlorpropamide (*Diabinese*)	
Digoxin, in dosages > 0.125 mg/d	Unless an atrial arrhythmia is being treated; high severity is considered if started within the past month
Disopyramide (*Norpace*)	
GI antispasmodics (belladonna alkaloids, clidinium, dicyclomine, hyoscyamine, propantheline)	Use for short periods (not over 7 d) on an intermittent basis (not more frequently than q 3 mo) does not require review by the surveyor
Meperidine, oral	If started within past month
Methyldopa	If started within past month
Pentazocine	
Ticlopidine	Review by the surveyor is not necessary in individuals who receive it because they have had a previous stroke or have evidence of stroke precursors (ie, TIAs) and cannot tolerate aspirin

The drug-diagnosis combinations specified in **Table 84** are considered "high severity" by CMS and should be considered potentially inappropriate for use in treating elderly persons.

Table 84. Diagnosis-Drug Combinations Considered "High Severity" by CMS		
Class or Drug	**Diagnosis**	**Comments**
Sedatives, hypnotics	COPD	Short-acting benzodiazepines are acceptable
NSAIDs	Active or recurrent gastritis, peptic ulcer disease, GERD	COX-2 inhibitors are not included on the list of NSAIDs
Metoclopramide	Seizures or epilepsy	
ASA, NSAIDs, dipyridamole, ticlopidine	Anticoagulation	
Anticholinergic drugs	BPH	
TCAs	Arrhythmias	If started within past month

The medications listed in **Table 85** are considered "low severity" by CMS and should be considered as potentially inappropriate in treating elderly patients.

Table 85. Drugs Considered "Low Severity" by CMS	
Class or Drug	**Comments**
Antihistamines	That is, with anticholinergic properties
Cyclandelate	
Digoxin, in dosages > 0.125 mg/d	Unless an atrial arrhythmia is being treated; high severity is considered if started within the past month
Diphenhydramine	Review by a surveyor is not necessary if used for a short time (not over 7 d) on an intermittent basis (not more frequently than q 3 mo) for allergies
Dipyridamole	
Ergot mesylates (eg, *Hydergine*)	
Indomethacin	Short-term use (eg, 1 wk) is considered acceptable for treatment of gouty arthritis
Meperidine, oral	If therapy longer than 1 mo
Muscle relaxants (eg, carisoprodol, chlorzoxazone, cyclobonzaprine, dantrolene, metaxalone, methocarbarnol, orphenadrine)	Use for short periods (not over 7 d) on an intermittent basis (not more frequently than q 3 mo) does not require review

The drug-diagnosis combinations specified in **Table 86** are considered "low severity" by the CMS and should be considered potentially inappropriate in all elderly patients.

Table 86. Diagnosis-Drug Combinations Considered "Low Severity" by CMS		
Class or Drug	**Diagnosis**	**Comments**
Corticosteroids	Diabetes mellitus	If started within past month
Potassium supplements or ASA (>325 mg/d)	Active or recurrent gastritis, peptic ulcer disease, or GERD	Use of potassium supplements to treat low potassium levels until they return to the normal range is permissible if prescriber determines that use of fresh fruits and vegetables or other dietary supplementation is not adequate or possible
Antipsychotics	Seizures or epilepsy	Treatment of acute psychosis for 72 h or less is permissible
Narcotic drugs, including propoxyphene	BPH	Review by the surveyor is not necessary if use is for short duration (7 d or less) on an intermittent basis (once q 3 mo) for symptoms of an acute, self-limiting condition
Bladder relaxants (flavoxate, oxybutynin, bethanechol)	BPH	Review by the surveyor is not necessary if use is for short duration (7 d or less) on an intermittent basis (once q 3 mo) for symptoms of an acute, self-limiting condition
Anticholinergic antihistamines, GI antispasmodics, anticholinergic antidepressants, and narcotic drugs (including propoxyphene)	Constipation	Constipation can be worsened Review by the surveyor is not necessary if use is for short duration (7 d or less) on an intermittent basis (once q 3 mo) for symptoms of an acute self-limiting condition
Antiparkinson medications	Constipation	Constipation can be worsened
Decongestants, theophylline, methylphenidate, SSRI antidepressants and desipramine, MAOIs, β-agonists	Insomnia	Insomnia can be worsened

IMPORTANT
TELEPHONE NUMBERS AND WEB SITES

General Aging

AGS Foundation for Health in Aging	www.healthinaging.org	(212) 755-6810
American Association of Retired Persons	www.aarp.org	(800) 424-3410
American Geriatrics Society	www.americangeriatrics.org	(212) 308-1414
American Medical Directors Association	www.amda.com	(800) 876-2632
American Society of Consultant Pharmacists	www.ascp.com	(800) 355-2727
Assisted Living Federation of America	www.alfa.org	(703) 691-8100
Children of Aging Parents	www.caps4caregivers.org	(800) 227-7294
CDC National Prevention Information Network	www.cdcnpin.org	(800) 458-5231
Family Caregiver Alliance	www.caregiver.org	(800) 445-8106
Medicare Hotline	www.medicare.gov	(800) MEDICARE
National Adult Day Services Association	www.nadsa.org	(866) 890-7357
National Council on the Aging	www.ncoa.org	(202) 479-1200
National Institute on Aging	www.nia.nih.gov	(800) 222-2225

Elder Abuse

National Center on Elder Abuse	www.elderabusecenter.org	(202) 898-2586

End-of-Life

Last Acts	www.lastacts.org	(202) 296-8071
National Hospice & Palliative Care Organization	www.nhpco.org	
For hospice referral		(800) 658-8898

Specific Health Problems

Alzheimer's Association	www.alz.org	(800) 272-3900
Alzheimer's Disease Education & Referral Center	www.alzheimers.org	(800) 438-4380
American Academy of Ophthalmology	www.aao.org	(800) 222-3937
American Association for Geriatric Psychiatry	www.aagponline.org	(301) 654-7850
American Cancer Society, Inc.	www.cancer.org	(800) ACS-2345
American College of Obstetricians & Gynecologists	www.acog.com	(800) 673-8444
American Diabetes Association	www.diabetes.org	(800) DIABETES
American Foundation for the Blind	www.afb.org	(800) AFB-LINE
American Heart Association	www.americanheart.org	(800) AHA-USA1
American Lung Association	www.lungusa.org	(800) LUNG-USA
American Pain Society	www.ampainsoc.org	(847)-375-4715
American Parkinson Disease Association	www.apdaparkinson.com	(800) 223-2732
American Urological Association	www.auanet.org	(410) 727-1100
Arthritis Foundation	www.arthritis.org	(800) 283-7800
Better Hearing Institute	www.betterhearing.org	(800) EARWELL
Lighthouse International	www.lighthouse.org	(800) 829-0500
Meals On Wheels Association of America	www.projectmeal.org	(703) 548-5558
National Institute of Arthritis & Musculoskeletal & Skin Diseases	www.niams.nih.gov	(877) 22-NIAMS
National Association for Continence	www.nafc.org	(800) BLADDER
National Diabetes Information Clearinghouse	www.niddk.nih.gov/health/diabetes/ndic.htm	
National Digestive Disease Information Clearinghouse	www.niddk.nih.gov/health/digest/nddic.htm	(800) 860-8747
		(800) 891-5389
National Eye Institute	www.nei.nih.gov	(301) 496-5248
National Heart, Lung & Blood Institute	www.nhlbi.nih.gov	(301) 592-8573

National Institute of Mental Health	www.nimh.nih.gov	(800) 421-4211
National Institute of Neurological Disorders & Stroke	www.ninds.nih.gov	(800) 352-9424
National Institute on Deafness & Other Communication Disorders	www.nidcd.nih.gov	TTY: (800) 241-1055; (800) 241-1044
National Kidney & Urologic Diseases Information Clearinghouse	www.niddk.nih.gov/health/kidney/nkudic.htm	(800) 891-5390
National Osteoporosis Foundation	www.nof.org	(800) 223-9994
National Parkinson Foundation	www.parkinson.org	(800) 327-4545
Self Help for Hard of Hearing People	www.shhh.org	TTY: (301) 657-2249; (301) 657-2248
Sexuality Information & Education Council of the US	www.siecus.org	(212) 819-9770
The Simon Foundation for Continence	www.simonfoundation.org	(800) 23-SIMON

Page references followed by *t* and *f* indicate tables and figures, respectively.
Trade names are in *italics*.

Page references followed by *t* and *f* indicate tables and figures, respectively.
Trade names are in *italics*.

Page references followed by *t* and *f* indicate tables and figures, respectively.
Trade names are in *italics*.

Page references followed by *t* and *f* indicate tables and figures, respectively.
Trade names are in *italics*.

Page references followed by *t* and *f* indicate tables and figures, respectively.
Trade names are in *italics*.

Page references followed by *t* and *f* indicate tables and figures, respectively.
Trade names are in *italics*.

Page references followed by *t* and *f* indicate tables and figures, respectively.
Trade names are in *italics*.

Page references followed by *t* and *f* indicate tables and figures, respectively.
Trade names are in *italics*.

Page references followed by *t* and *f* indicate tables and figures, respectively.
Trade names are in *italics*.

Page references followed by *t* and *f* indicate tables and figures, respectively. Trade names are in *italics*.

Page references followed by t and f indicate tables and figures, respectively.
Trade names are in *italics*.

Page references followed by *t* and *f* indicate tables and figures, respectively.
Trade names are in *italics*.

Page references followed by *t* and *f* indicate tables and figures, respectively.
Trade names are in *italics*.

Page references followed by *t* and *f* indicate tables and figures, respectively.
Trade names are in *italics*.

Page references followed by *t* and *f* indicate tables and figures, respectively.
Trade names are in *italics*.

Page references followed by *t* and *f* indicate tables and figures, respectively.
Trade names are in *italics*.

Page references followed by *t* and *f* indicate tables and figures, respectively.
Trade names are in *italics*.

Page references followed by *t* and *f* indicate tables and figures, respectively.
Trade names are in *italics*.

Page references followed by *t* and *f* indicate tables and figures, respectively.
Trade names are in *italics*.

Page references followed by *t* and *f* indicate tables and figures, respectively.
Trade names are in *italics*.

Page references followed by *t* and *f* indicate tables and figures, respectively.
Trade names are in *italics*.

Page references followed by *t* and *f* indicate tables and figures, respectively.
Trade names are in *italics*.

Page references followed by *t* and *f* indicate tables and figures, respectively.
Trade names are in *italics*.

Page references followed by *t* and *f* indicate tables and figures, respectively.
Trade names are in *italics*.

Page references followed by *t* and *f* indicate tables and figures, respectively.
Trade names are in *italics*.

ABOUT THE AMERICAN GERIATRICS SOCIETY

Founded in 1942, the American Geriatrics Society (AGS) is the leading clinical society devoted to the care of older adults. The AGS promotes high quality, comprehensive, and accessible care for America's older population, including those who are chronically ill and disabled. The organization provides leadership to health care professionals, policy makers, and the public by developing, implementing, and advocating programs in patient care, research, professional and public education, and public policy.

Its 6000 members include primary care physicians, geriatricians, geropsychiatrists, nurse practitioners, social workers, physician assistants, physical therapists, pharmacists, and others from the United States and around the world who are dedicated to improving the health, independence, and quality of life of the older population.

The AGS has long championed efforts to expand the national work force of clinicians with the specialized knowledge and skills to care for our aging population. Since the early 1990s, with funding from the John A. Hartford Foundation of New York City, the AGS has worked effectively to increase geriatrics expertise among subspecialists in internal medicine, practicing primary care physicians, and nonprimary care specialists.

In 1999, the AGS reached beyond its traditional role as a professional medical society and launched the **Foundation for Health in Aging (FHA)**. The FHA aims to build a bridge between the research/practice of geriatrics health care professionals and the public, and to advocate on behalf of older adults regarding issues of wellness and preventive care, self-responsibility and independence, and connections to family and community. For more information about FHA initiatives, please visit the Foundation Web site at http://www.healthinaging.org.

Current Major Publications and Programs of the AGS Include:
Journal of the American Geriatrics Society—rated in the top three of the ISI Science Citation Index for geriatrics and gerontology publications.

Annals of Long-Term Care: Clinical Care and Aging—This journal presents the highest quality clinical reviews, analysis, and opinions that impact the present and future of long-term care, and is the premier source of information for professionals in the long-term care market.

Clinical Geriatrics—This journal focuses on both the clinical and practical issues related to the treatment and management of older persons.

Geriatrics Review Syllabus: A Core Curriculum in Geriatric Medicine—the ground-breaking self-assessment, continuing education program for primary care providers and a premier source of clinically relevant information in geriatric medicine, now in its 5th edition.

Geriatrics At Your Fingertips—a comprehensive pocket-sized reference to clinical geriatrics that provides up-to-date, practical information on the evaluation and management of diseases and disorders most common to elderly people. Updated annually. Visit the *Fingertips* web site at http://www.geriatricsatyourfingertips.org.

Geriatrics Review Syllabus for Specialists—Derived from both *Geriatrics At Your Fingertips* and the *Geriatrics Review Syllabus,* this textbook focuses on the surgical approach to the elderly patient.

Public Education Publications from the Foundation for Health in Aging—*Patient Education Forums* provide answers to commonly asked questions on a variety of geriatrics topics. *Eldercare at Home* is an extensive guide for families involved in providing care for older relatives who want to remain at home. Information on these and other public education programs is available on the Foundation Web site.

AGS Newsletter and AGS Web site (http://www.americangeriatrics.org)—excellent sources of information on AGS activities and programs, noteworthy news, public policy issues, career opportunities in geriatrics, and much more.

Policy Position Statements and Clinical Practice Guidelines—In its Clinical Practice Guidelines series, the AGS has recently released the updated guideline "The Management of Persistent Pain in Older Persons" as a supplement to the June 2002 issue of the *Journal of the American Geriatrics Society.* The AGS publishes position statements, papers, and guidelines to bring important issues in geriatrics education, research, clinical practice, and public policy to the attention of those working in the field, including policy makers, legislators, people in the health care industry, clinicians, and others.

The AGS Annual Scientific Meeting—the premier forum for the latest information on clinical geriatrics, research on aging and health, problems of older adults, and innovative models in health care delivery as well as teaching in geriatrics.

The Geriatrics Recognition Award—awarded to recognize physicians and nurses who are committed to advancing their geriatrics knowledge in order to provide better care to older adults.

The AGS Awards Program—includes the following: the Edward Henderson Award and State-of-the-Art Lecture; AGS Clinician of the Year; AGS/Merck New Investigator Awards; Pfizer/AGS Postdoctoral Fellowship Awards; Dennis W. Jahnigen Memorial Award; the Nascher/Manning Award; the Outstanding Scientific Clinical Investigator Award; the Edward Henderson Student Award; and the AGS Student Research Award.

Special Projects in Professional Education/Outreach are funded by foundations and industry sponsors.

If you would like further information about the AGS, please contact us at:

The American Geriatrics Society
Empire State Building
350 5th Avenue, Suite 801
New York, NY 10118
http://www.americangeriatrics.org
or
Call the AGS toll free at
1-800-247-4779
or
Send e-mail
info.amger@americangeriatrics.org

GERIATRICS *At Your* FINGERTIPS
2003, 5th Edition
(ISBN 140510337X)
From the American Geriatrics Society

A guide to the evaluation and management of the diseases and disorders that most commonly affect older persons.

Portable, Practical, Fully Indexed, and Up-to-Date!

Send completed order form with payment to:

Blackwell Publishing
c/o AIDC
PO Box 20
Williston, VT 05495-0020

For fast service
Call: 800-216-2522
Fax: 800-864-7626
E-mail: orders@aidcvt.com

Please send me _____ copies of *Geriatrics At Your Fingertips*, 2003, 5th Edition @ $11.95 each

Subtotal   _____

Sales Tax (MA, VT, CA, NY and Canada)   _____

Shipping & Handling   _____
(No. Amer: $5.00 + $1.00 ea additional
Overseas: $8.00 + $1.00 ea additional)

TOTAL   _____

To order quantities of 25 or greater please contact our special sales department at 800-759-6102 X8341.

Method of Payment: _____ Check or money order payable to Blackwell

_____ MasterCard   _____VISA   _____AMEX

Card Number _____ Exp.Date _____

Signature _____

Shipping Instructions (must be complete)

Name: _____
Address: _____
City: _____State: _____ Zip: _____
Phone: _____
E-mail Address: _____

GAYF2003

Your request places you on the Blackwell e-alert electronic mailing list. You will be among the first in your discipline to find out about new releases, special offers and textbook announcements from Blackwell. After you receive your first e-alert, you have the option of canceling the service at any time. Prices subject to change without notice.